Working BRAIMemory

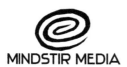

MINDSTIR MEDIA

Working Brain Memory

Copyright © 2020 by Jaime Leal Sotelo, PhD. All rights reserved.

Published by Mindstir Media, LLC
45 Lafayette Rd | Suite 181| North Hampton, NH 03862 | USA
1.800.767.0531 | www.mindstirmedia.com

Printed in the United States of America
ISBN-13: 978-1-7356910-3-9

Working BRAIMemory

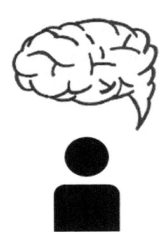

Jaime Leal Sotelo, PhD

Contents

PART II - THE HOW

50+ INTERACTIVE WORKING MEMORY CONTENT BASED ACTIVITIES

PART I
THE WHY

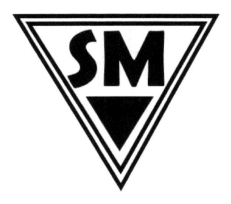

Super Memory, Our Hero

Imagine you are driving on the freeway, and then all of a sudden, you witness a truck hitting a car. The truck left the scene, but you had a few seconds to see the truck's license plate. Since you are a nice and considerate person, you memorized the truck plate to help the unfortunate driver of the car as a witness when the police arrive.

Memorize the following license plate:

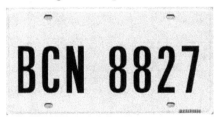

The average brain stores around seven pieces of information for approximately thirty seconds. This information will be lost if there is not any attempt to retain the material. To preserve the data in the brain for a longer period of time, it will be necessary to re-expose the brain to the information and establish a maintenance process for the input.

CHALLENGE 1

Now say the truck plate.

CHALLENGE 2

Let's put our brains to work for a little bit.

Try to say the numbers from the truck plate in order from least to greatest.

Now try to say the letters in alphabetical order.

Recall is the action of remembering something already learned. As you were saying the truck plate to yourself, you were bringing back stored information from your memory.

The previous task of memorizing the truck plate is an example of how you will be challenging your working memory in several other tests in this book. First, you will receive stimuli like the truck plate for a few seconds. Afterward, you will have a distractor, such as the explanation of the seven pieces of information that you previously read, to divert your brain from the truck plate. Then, you will recall the material retained, in other words, repeating the truck plate. Finally, you will receive the challenge of manipulating the information in your brain; in this case, you had to organize the numbers from least to greatest and letters in alphabetical order. Researchers found that stimulating working memory provides advantages that go beyond memory, but produces benefits in academic performance (Holmes et al., 2009).

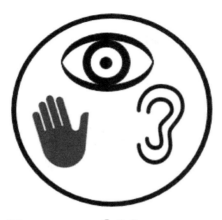

Types of Memory

In 1960, Richard Atkinson and Richard Shiffrin proposed a model for memory; they claimed that the information we receive comes from the environment through our sensory registers, and memory such as iconic, echoic, or haptic, receive it. Then, this information goes to a short-term storage system called working memory. If the information is relevant to our brain and rehearsed constantly, it would be stored in long-term memory.

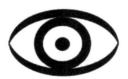

Visual or Iconic Memory

Get ready because you will see a shape in the form of a cross. Look at the white dot in the center for about ten seconds. Then, close your eyes and count the seconds until the shape vanishes while you have your eyes shut.

Ready?

Now, look at the white point at the center of the cross for about ten seconds, and then close your eyes.

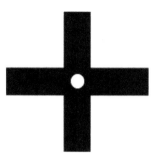

How many seconds did you count before the shape vanished while you have your eyes shut?

_____seconds.

You probably counted a few seconds, but Swedish investigator Segner found that iconic memory is around one-tenth of a second. This is our sensory visual or iconic memory at work. To make a point about iconic memory, place your hand right in front of your face and move it right and left continuously. You will see that your fingers leave a kind of faded or blurred image. When you move your hand that fast, there is an interruption of the scene for a short period giving the retina the opportunity to be refreshed before it goes to the next scene. Iconic memory serves as a visual support to our senses to input information into our brains.

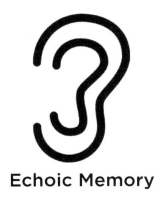

Echoic Memory

In a moment, you will be asked to close your eyes and register the last sound you heard in your memory. While you have your eyes closed, you will point at the direction where you heard the last sound.

Ready? Now close your eyes and point at the direction of the last sound you heard.

Being able to recall the direction of the sound is part of the echoic memory. It is also important to say that your ears do not receive the sound waves instantly, but there is a delay until the sound travels from the source of the message into your ears. It could have taken a fraction of a second until it reached your ears. The brain is so intuitive that it closes the gap between what it observes and what it hears. For example, if you hear me clapping, there is a delay in sound. What you see is immediate, but the sound of the clapping did not reach your ear at the same time. The brain coordinated this gap so you could see and hear simultaneously. It is important to close your eyes, leaving your sense of hearing in charge of the situation; in this manner, the effects of echoic memory could have more lasting results than iconic memory.

In the task of memorizing the previous truck plate, you have to look at the numbers and letters for a few seconds and then recall them. It is easier to recall more digits if you heard them or say them to yourself.

In serial recall, auditory presentation yields an advantage over visual presentation alone (Cowan et al. 2002). Listening to information has a great impact on our memory and more if you inhibit your vision by closing your eyes. Further, researchers claim that auditory input has an advantaged access to cognitive systems (Salamé and Baddeley, 1982; McLeod and Posner, 1984).

Think of one three-word instruction that you give to your students.

Examples:

Sharpen your pencil

Read your book

Bring your notebook

Raise your hand

Write your student's instruction here:

_____   _____   _____

Echoic memory refers to the resonance in which the last sounding stimuli would be repeating in your brain. Whatever the last piece of information received was, this is what you will keep in your brain.

Let's say that you give an instruction to your students, such as, "Place your pencil in your desk." Since *desk* was the last word you said, *desk* would be echoing in students' brains. Since the word *desk* is relevant, students would have more probability to follow this instruction.

What about if you say, "Place your pencil in your desk, and follow the rule,"? Since *rule* was the last word heard, it would be echoing in the students' brains. What are the probabilities that students follow the instruction?

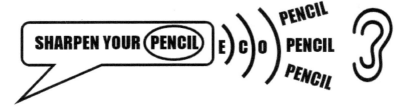

The word pencil would be echoing in students' ears.

Now go back to the list of instructions and circle the last word that would be the echoing sound in the students' brains. Next time, when you say an instruction, plan to take into account echoic memory.

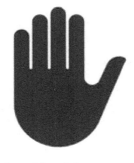

Haptic Memory

Another way to get input from the environment is through the sense of touch called **haptic memory**. This is mostly used to assess the degree of strength used to grab an object. The level of strength used to grab a pencil will be different than to grasp a brick. Have you tried to cut a sheet of paper using scissors? What about trying to cut cardboard using the same scissors? Your sense of touch allows you to feel and evaluate how much more force you need to use to cut different materials. Your brain detects patterns and uses this knowledge to apply the force necessary in the situation at hand.

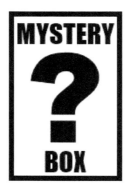

**Students would describe a hidden object
through the sense of touch.**

In the mystery box activity, an object is placed inside a box. Students must guess what the object is via touch. This enhances haptic memory since there are no other senses involved. This task allows inhibiting the sense of vision and leaves the sense of touch in charge of discovering the item inside.

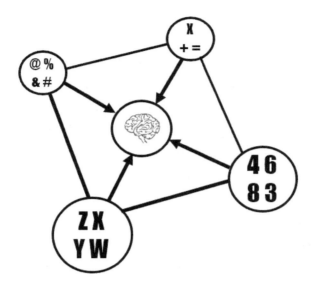

The Power of Information

What is the forecasted temperature for tomorrow for your area?

_____

List three decisions that you would make knowing this information.

1. _____

2. _____

3. _____

Certainly, the more information we have, the better decisions we can make. Undoubtedly, the brain holds a massive quantity of information in storage ready to use. The accessibility of information is essential. If you can access the right information at the right moment, you can respond to situations effectively. Knowing more puts us at an advantage over others. How can working memory help in accessing more information? If you expand your memory, it will be like a domino effect in which one thing topples others.

Let's say that you can store more information in your memory than others do. If you practice expanding your working memory, it will exponentially increase the information you have at hand to use at any time. Working memory and long-term memory work together as a team. Working memory requests information from long-term memory and acts as the hand that picks up the folder from a file cabinet. Working memory is selective because it only grabs what it needs or what is available to solve the situation at hand. It is also important how quickly this information is obtained from the file cabinet (long-term memory). An expanded working memory will help us have better access to long-term memory since they communicate with each other to resolve the issue at hand. An expanded working memory is faster, more efficient, and gives a precise response when it is necessary.

Technology has led us not to rely on memory since we have computers that can store huge amounts of information. We can even find information on the internet whenever we need it. On the one hand, technology has helped, but on the other hand, it has made us lethargic. In the book *The Smartest Kids in the World* by Amanda Ripley, Polish students were using mental math in the classroom, and it seemed to come automatically after a while. The brain should be doing that simple automatic math instead of relying on calculators, as some schools allow. Working memory is our brain's calculator and manipulator of information, and the more it is used, the more capacity it builds.

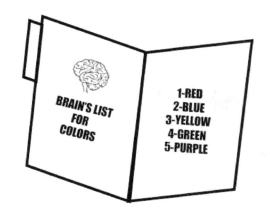

Accessing Information

Let's do the next exercise. In your mind, place the following months in alphabetical order.

November

December

January

February

March

April

Now think of a color. _____

Now think of a tool. _____

Did you pick either of these tools?

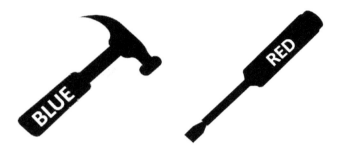

The activity of ordering the months by alphabetical order was not relevant at all. It was just a distraction to keep your brain busy and give immediate access to your long-term memory. Imagine long-term memory as a file cabinet. Inside, you have many folders, and in each folder, you have lists of items. The color you mentioned first is the item you have first in your list. Why is it first? There are many possibilities. Maybe this is your favorite color, or you have seen this color painted in your room for so long that it is ingrained in your mind and took the first place in your memory's list of colors. The same effect happens with the tool. If you said screwdriver, it might be the most common tool you rely on when you need to fix something and that is why it was first in your list of tools. People have different responses depending on individual experiences.

Look at the following statement. Answer with the first response that comes to your mind.

Say the color of a bear.

Answer_____

Most people will say brown or black. The color black is what most of the regular bears are, but what about the polar bear, which is white or the panda bear, which is black and white? Again, the first response is what is first in our list of colors for bears.

Here are other examples you can try.

Say a sea creature.
Say a type of a monkey.
Say a kind of car.

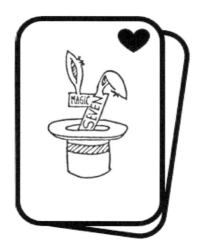

Magic Number 7

Try to memorize the following number.

9042658

Now, close the book and say the number.

If you said them all correctly, you are average. Most people can manage about seven digits. You will be more successful memorizing if you verbalize the numbers rather than just trying to memorize them quietly. Articulating and listening to the numbers helps the memory to register the information briefly in auditory memory.

Another strategy to memorize is grouping them in chunks of two or three numbers with a little pause in between the groups. If you add some rhythm such as the way poets use rhyme and rhythm, the information is absorbed even more effectively.

Use the keypad below to help you ingrain the numbers using another brain pathway.

9042658

Now, say the number using the keypad.

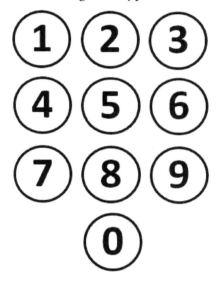

Now, say only the even numbers.

4268

In the first request, you recalled the numbers. In the second request, you manipulated the information. You probably noticed that the recall task was easier, but it took more time during the manipulation of the information, which is one of the functions of working memory. In other words, working memory is equal to mental manipulation, mental calculation, mental judging, or mental agility.

Your brain finds different strategies like forming a pattern in the keypad to make sense of the information and make it easier to memorize. Sometimes it is necessary to use all the resources you have available to store information in different pathways in your brain—visual, auditory, or using movements.

Now close the book and dial the number in the air. Is it easier? I bet it was. Here is where associations come in handy. We get a number out of nothing and use something familiar like our number pad to memorize it.

This is how you probably visualize the number in your brain using a keypad with arrows simulating the patterns of numbers.

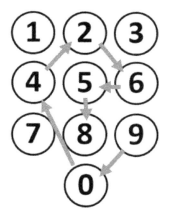

Here are some other strategies you could use:

1. Chunk the information–Placing numbers in groups helps to make sense of numbers and prevents an overload of information.

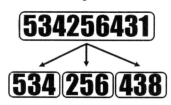

2. Associate the numbers with a date. You decide the chunk of numbers you want and the association you could form with it. Since numbers are abstract, chunking and associating numbers in pairs is the most useful way to retain the information.

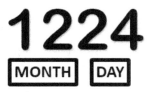

3. Associate two digits with an item or a concept, just like the example below.

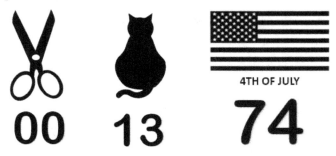

4. Make a story with the numbers. Assign them to an established item and create a story. A visualization of a foolish story will make it more memorable.

On the fourth of July a black cat chase me with scissors

In 1956, George Miller coined the term "The Magical Number Seven, Plus or Minus Two," asserting that individuals can hold around seven pieces of information in their brains for a few seconds establishing a fixed capacity for retaining information. The good news is that working memory is not fixed. Studies have found that as we grow up, working memory develops and increases (Gathercole and Alloway, 2007). The brain's capacity is not fixed, and its adaptable plasticity allows for improvement via targeted cognitive training exercises in areas such as **speed of processing** (Ball et al., 2002), **attention** (Green and Bavelier, 2003; Bherer et al., 2008), **working memory** (Klingberg, 2010, Wykes et al., 2002; Valenzuela et al., 2003; Westerberg et al., 2007; Schmiedek et al., 2010) and **fluid intelligence** (Jaeggi et al., 2008).

**Children can juggle only 2-3 pieces
of information in their brains.**

Adults 20s-30s hold 6 pieces of information.

Adults 40-up hold 5 pieces of information.

By exposing students to content-based working memory activities, we target those students with poor working memory capacity and help them develop it. Students with average working memory can extend it, and students with exceptional working memory capacity maintain their ability.

Student's Actual Working Memory Capacity	Yields of Exposing Students to Working Memory Activities
Poor working memory	Develop working memory
Average working memory	Extend working memory
Exceptional working memory	Maintain working memory

Ross and Tracy Alloway (2013) found in their lifespan studies that adults in their twenties and thirties can hold six pieces of information, and children can manage only two to three. People in their forties had the disadvantage of working memory decline in which managing information is reduced to five pieces representing a 20% decline compared to their twenties and thirties. However, do not panic. As people age, that decrease in information capacity is compensated for with more efficient retrieval of accumulated knowledge (experience). Older brains manage to compensate for the decline using strategies and recruiting more neurons for a specific task than those of younger people. In addition, older brains have to work harder and have to use more brain areas to get the job done.

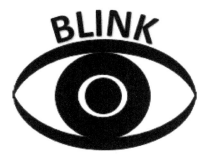

With a Blink of an Eye-Fovea

The fovea is the high-resolution center in our eye. Without it, everything around our fovea would look blurred.

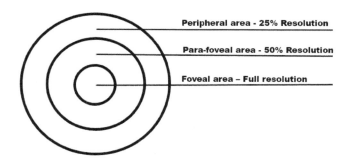

Peripheral area - 25% Resolution

Para-foveal area - 50% Resolution

Foveal area – Full resolution

To experience your fovea's visual acuteness, stare at the bolded "**o**" letter in the middle of the following word. Do not move your eyes. You will feel tempted to roll your eyes away but keep them fixed on the letter "**o**" and count how many letters you can read clearly on either side of the letter.

Ready?

Pneumonoultramicrosc**o**picsilicovolcanokoniosis

You can place a mark on either side of the word to record your fovea acuity.

Left_____ Right_____ = _____ Total letters

How many letters were you able to see?

Now you know your fovea acuity capacity.

The previous word is the longest word in any of the major English language dictionaries. It is a lung disease that develops from inhaling silica volcano particles.

Most people report that they can only read about five to seven letters on either side. So, to read a page of text, even though the entire page falls on your retina, you have to move your eyes across the page successively fixating on different words at a time to be able to see them clearly enough to read them.

The fovea occupies only one percent of our retinal size but takes up to fifty percent of the visual cortex in the brain. The fovea is the source of most of the information we receive due to its clarity on details. Eyes need to move around the item under observation, so the fovea absorbs the specifics with accuracy. We can assume that individuals in the blink of an eye have access to only five to seven characters in high resolution and everything else in the surroundings would be blurred.

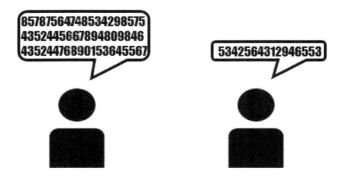

Working Memory:
The Brain's Scrap Paper

You are driving in an unknown city, and your cell phone is dead, so you cannot access your GPS. You have no other option than to stop in the convenience store and ask for directions to reach your destination.

Here are the directions you received from the store clerk. Try to memorize them.

1. Go south and turn at the next right.
2. Keep driving three blocks and then turn right.
3. Take the next left.
4. You will find it on your right in the middle of the block.

Cover the instructions and trace the directions on the map.

You are at the star.

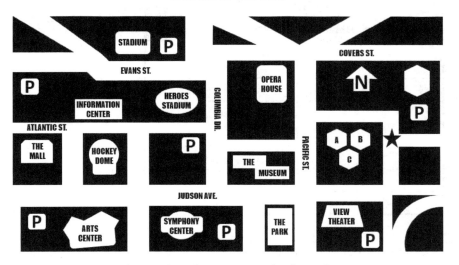

What is the place you are looking for?

_____

If you arrived at the information center, you have a great memory.

Following directions is a typical working memory test and more challenging when you only have a quick chance to hear the directions one time. In this activity, the instructions were shown for a short time, assuming that the store clerk did not have the opportunity to repeat the instructions as many times as you needed because they are busy working. Then, you have to recall the information to reach your destination. This is a great way to challenge your working memory.

Age	Number of instructions according to age	School Grade
5-6	2 instructions	K-1st
7-9	3 instructions	2-4
10-12	4 instructions	5-7
13-15	5 instructions	8-10
16-39	6 instructions	11 and over
40-49	5 instructions	
50-59	4 instructions	
60-69	3 instructions	

Sometimes at work, I have something that I do not want to forget, so I write it on a Post-it note and keep it in my shirt pocket. When I arrive home and see the note, I remember to do something with the information after I see it, then I throw away the Post-it note since it served its purpose. I see working memory as a Post-it note, which holds the information for a moment until I do something with it.

Another way I see working memory is to think of the brain as a whiteboard on which we can write information in our minds, use it, and then erase it, leaving the blank space for other information. There are different brain whiteboard sizes in which you can keep writing information until you run out of space. Working memory works the same way. There are different capacities, but it can get clogged with an overload of information.

Look at your working memory like your own mental scratch paper. When people take a test, sometimes they are allowed to have some scratch paper for quick notes or calculations during the test. Once the test is finished, the scratch paper is no longer needed, but it was important to completing the test. Working memory functions the same way by storing information or making those mental calculations at the moment you need them.

Working memory coordinates with long-term memory with a component that Baddeley called the episodic buffer, which integrates information from both parties. The access of pieces of information depends on the route of the connection. It will be easier to access the information if this connection has been used more often. Let's imagine that you are trying to find a file about marketing on your computer, but you do not remember where it is. You start looking through your folders to see if there is any connection between the different folders and this marketing file. Finally, you see one folder named advertising. You click on this advertising folder, and you see a list of files but now, where is the marketing file? Access to this information is not direct; instead, there are many obstacles in the way. The brain works the same way; some connections are more accessible than others. Practicing working memory activities will reinforce those connections and pathways in the brain to make them more accessible.

Understanding Working Memory

One of the most accepted definitions of working memory is Baddeley's theoretical model (1993). Baddeley defined working memory as the limited-capacity storage system involved in the maintenance and manipulation of information over a short period of time. In the earlier truck license plate activity at the beginning of the book, the information was not manipulated in the brain but retained for a few seconds until it was necessary to be recalled. Working memory goes a step further than just recalling the information, but manipulating it, doing something with the material retained.

Baddeley's working memory theoretical model consists of four elements. The *phonological loop* is in charge of maintaining the auditory information. The *visuospatial sketchpad* is responsible for visual and spatial information. The third component is the *central executive system*. This part of working memory holds, manipulates, coordinates, and sometimes when necessary, inhibits information. Finally, the *episodic buffer* takes information from the working memory and long-term memory and integrates it.

Researchers have described the two critical functions of working memory: retention and manipulation of information. Tracy and Ross Alloway (2013) defined working memory as the conscious processing of information. Information is consciously stored in your mind and can be manipulated by making calculations or making decisions with it. Working memory, the cognitive system responsible for the temporary storage and manipulation of information, is crucial for maintaining focused behavior in practical situations (Kane et al., 2007).

Behind your forehead, on the other side of your skull, you will find the prefrontal cortex. In this precise location, the most important cognitive functions of the brain are processed, such as problem-solving, making decisions, and other cognitive functions. The prefrontal cortex is the part of the brain that houses working memory.

Location of working memory in the brain

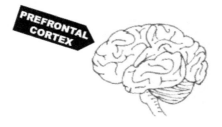

Researchers using brain scans have located working memory mainly in the frontal lobes (Stuss and Alexander, 2000; Pennington and Ozonoff, 1996). The prefrontal cortex is where most of the working memory functions are located; however, there are other areas in the brain that support or help during the processing of working memory. The areas of the brain where working memory functions as a whole memory network are the prefrontal, temporal, and parietal (Baddeley and Logie, 1999). The location of working memory, according to Tracy and Ross Alloway (2013) in their book, *Working Memory Advantage* is in the prefrontal cortex, hippocampus, amygdala, intraparietal sulcus, and Broca's area.

Area of the brain supporting working memory	Function
Hippocampus	The hippocampus is where your long-term memories are stored. Working memory depends on the hippocampus to pull important information associated with the task at hand. The hippocampus supports the process of providing stored background knowledge to make connections with new information.
Amygdala	The amygdala is where the emotions are located. Working memory helps to control and inhibit emotions to be able to perform a working memory task. When working memory is functioning, the amygdala is put to rest, and likewise, working memory is put into rest when the amygdala is in action.
Intraparietal Sulcus	The intraparietal sulcus supports working memory by providing the answers to mental math. It is where calculations are processed. When researchers directed an electrical current to the intraparietal sulcus to inhibit this part of the brain, individuals were unable to make simple calculations. Research has found that brain activity in the intraparietal sulcus predicted arithmetic performance (Dumontheil, and Klingberg, 2012). In another study, Rotzer (2009) found that children with low math ability have lower levels of brain activity in the right intraparietal sulcus.
Broca's Area	Broca's area is where language comprehension and verbal fluency are located in the brain. Working memory relies on Broca's area when you forget your shopping list, and you try to remember it mentally.

Within the framework of working memory, a simple task related to the phonological loop is when people are verbally introduced with a series of numbers and are asked to recall the numbers in the order presented.

9874345

A task for the visuospatial sketchpad is when participants are presented with a shape for few seconds. Then when the shape is removed, participants are asked to recall the location of the shaded squares.

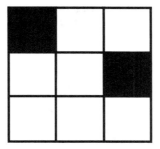

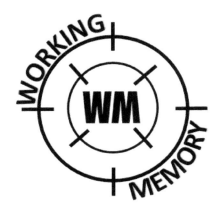

Why is Working Memory Important?

To understand why working memory is important, it is necessary to embrace the cognitive and academic benefits it provides. Years of research have demonstrated that working memory is important for different functions. Working memory is essential for complex cognitive processes such as spoken and written language, comprehension, mental arithmetic, reasoning, and problem-solving (e.g. Baddeley, 1986).

Further, research has shown that working memory is essential for learning and education. There is an important link between working memory and vocabulary acquisition (Gathercole and Martin 2011). Some fundamental functions of working memory also affect reading (Gathercole and Aloway 2008). There is also a critical relationship to arithmetic and mathematics (Arndt et al., 2013; Bull and Scerif 2001; DeStefano and LeFevre 2004; Mayringer and Wimmer, 2000; Siegel and Ryan, 1989; Swanson and Kim, 2007); and comprehension (Cain et al., 2004; Nation et al., 1999).

Working memory is necessary for learning a second language. There is a specific link between verbal and short-term memory and language acquisition in both the native and foreign language (Baddeley et al., 1998; Gathercole et al., 1997; Service and Craik, 1993; Service and Kohonen, 1995).

Working memory is a better predictor for academic success than IQ. Tracy and Ross Alloway (2009) found that working memory can predict scores of students with a 95 percent accuracy. In their study, they recruited two hundred kindergarten students and tested their working memory and IQ. They found that working memory was a better predictor of success in school than IQ. In another study with gifted students, they found that students with high IQ, but poor working memory, are more likely to be underachievers while those with high IQ and high working memory are more likely to succeed.

According to Tracy Alloway, IQ is closely linked to parental income. On the other hand, working memory is not linked to parental income, leveling the field for those who are economically disadvantaged. In addition, the more educated the parent, the higher the IQ of their children. This is likely due to more exposure to experiences like traveling, afterschool activities, and more opportunities. Having a higher IQ does not guarantee a well-developed working memory.

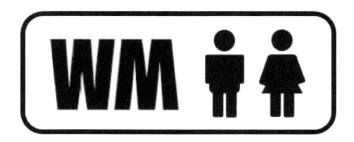

Working Memory and Gender

A meta-analysis study by Hill et al., (2014) showed consistent working memory activation networks across genders. However, there are some other differences in gender brain activation. Females activated the amygdala, hippocampus, and the right inferior frontal gyrus. The function of the amygdala is to generate memories related to emotions. The hippocampus is known for the storage of long-term memories. The right inferior frontal gyrus plays an important role in response inhibition. Males activated the parietal regions, which processes sensory information in the brain.

When working memory is deconstructed into verbal and spatial, gender differences arise. Females displayed fluency in verbal (Lewin et al., 2001) and writing skills. Males demonstrate fluency in mathematical (Lynn and Irwing, 2008), and spatial working memory activities (Kaufman, 2007; Lejbak et al., 2011; Masters and Sanders, 1993; Nordvik and Amponsah, 1998).

Females	Males
• Brain networks activation in the amygdala (emotions), hippocampus (long-term memory), and the right inferior frontal gyrus. • Displayed fluency in verbal and writing skills.	• Brain networks activation in the parietal regions. • Demonstrated fluency in mathematics and spatial working memory.

A study by Goldstein et al., 2005, suggests that females and males utilize different brain networks or strategies to solve complex problems in working memory. Based on gender differences, it is critical to teach female and male students using methods that correspond to their cognitive processes.

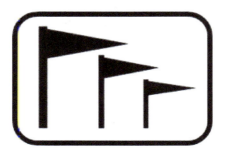

Red Flags

A teacher gives the following instruction to the classroom: "Please get your math journal out. Write your name, date, and the objective of the day." Brandon listened to all the instructions and got a journal out but not the math journal. When he finally found his pencil, he can write his name, but he did not write the date or the objective of the day. Brandon represents students with poor working memory. Studies found that 10% of students, ages 7 to 8 years old, have the working memory of a 4-year-old. Another study suggests that 15% of typical learners in the classroom have low working memory (Holmes et al., 2010). A student with poor working memory is at a disadvantage and would not meet the academic requirements of the classroom. Challenging students with working memory activities will provide them with the tools to be successful in cognitive and academic assignments. Some of the effects of poor working memory are that students start an assignment, but later lose track of important information affecting the flow of the assignment. This could lead to daydreaming, distractions, or simply giving up on the assignment. It is crucial to know when this situation happens, so adequate interventions are provided. Some of those behaviors could be avoided if an effective working memory practice process is implemented.

Some "red flags" that might indicate poor working memory
• Difficulty following lengthy directions
• Difficulty understanding long spoken sentences
• Trouble staying on topic in conversations
• Trouble with multistep math problems
• Difficulty with reading comprehension
• Struggles with completing tasks
• Memory problems
• Low grades
• Poor learning skill

Children with a poor working memory typically struggle in these activities, and over time these learning failures disrupt the normal incremental process of acquiring skills and knowledge throughout the school years, leading to poor educational progress (Gathercole et al., 2006).

Studies have found that students with poor working memory have a disadvantage in a range of cognitive activities, including remembering, following instructions, writing, and mental math.

Inattention and poor working memory are also highly connected. The children with low working memory are the ones we find staring out the window with their minds wandering (Kane et al., 2007) when tasks get too tough, and working memory gets overloaded.

Weak performance on arithmetic word problems is also a characteristic of poor verbal working memory (Swanson and Sachse-Lee, 2001).

Numerical information such as number representation, place value, and arithmetic are closely related to visual-spatial memory (Geary, 1990; McLean and Hitch, 1999). Students with poor visuospatial memory would have less space to process relevant numerical information. Studies have shown a relationship between poor working memory and poor computational skills (Wilson and Swanson, 2001).

Additionally, students who struggle academically are three times more susceptible to have poor working memory and special education learners are six times more susceptible than average students (Holmes et al., 2010). What this tells us is that the majority of students who perform poorly in school, or who require additional support, have working memory deficits. These are the kids who become overloaded during regular classroom activities, such as those involving multi-step instructions and miss out on important learning opportunities (Gathercole and Alloway, 2008).

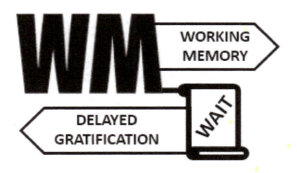

Working Memory and Delayed Gratification

Tracy Alloway (2013) specified that working memory acts as a conductor with three main functions: process, prioritize, and retain information. Working memory works as a conductor by selecting and holding important information to work with it. It also helps you to inhibit the information you do not need. Some advantages of working memory are that it helps you concentrate on what matters, make quick judgments, solve problems, learn more easily, and switch gears when something is not working. In stressful times, working memory helps you to inhibit the negative and work in the positive. Working memory helps in delaying gratification by making the best decision in the long-term instead of choosing the instant reward.

In 1968, psychologist Walter Mischel studied delayed gratification by offering marshmallows to more than 600 children between the ages of four and six. Then he told the children that he was going to leave the room for a few minutes, and if they could wait until he returned, they would get a second marshmallow. Children were instructed that if they could not wait, they could ring a bell, and he would return and let them eat the marshmallow. Most of the children ate the treat while a few others resisted the temptation and held out for the greater reward of two marshmallows.

We can see many features of working memory tasks in high-delayers such as keeping a greater reward in mind, ignoring distractions, diverting attention, planning and executing strategies. Some children used strategies such as hiding under the table, covering their eyes with their hands, turning their chairs the opposite way, or singing a song to keep them from being tempted to eat the marshmallow. The researchers followed up with the students several years later, and they compared their SAT scores. The amazing thing they found was those who delayed the gratification in the marshmallow test got the higher scores. Now high-delayer adults have found that their children were high-delayers too. They were able to resist the marshmallow for longer than their parents did. Those children who are high-delayers are able to control impulses and ignore temptations, which is a skill that working memory offers.

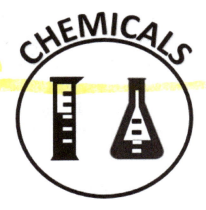

Working Memory Makes Us Happy

What makes you happy?_____

When people feel happy, there is a release of chemicals into the brain, such as dopamine and serotonin. When dopamine is released, a short-term feeling of joy is delivered to our brain and body. When serotonin is released, a sense of long-term happiness is delivered to the brain. Researchers discovered that brains in participants with high working memory produced more dopamine than those with low working memory.

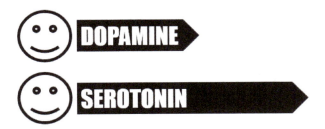

Dopamine provides a sense of happiness for a short time.
The release of serotonin boosts happiness long-term.

In another study, researchers found that participants performing a working memory task experience a greater release of serotonin than those who performed a non working memory task. Studies suggest that when individuals are challenged with working memory tasks, those good chemicals are released into the brain and make us feel good. Just being exposed to working memory challenges have the same effect on happiness, keeping those good chemicals coming.

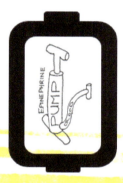

Another chemical that the brain produces is epinephrine (adrenaline), which is a stress chemical that sends blood to muscles so they are ready for action. The body in distress also releases cortisol, which is fuel in the form of sugar. A meta-analysis study has found that cortisol enhances inhibition (Shields et al., 2016). Both chemicals allow the body to react in fight-or-flight situations.

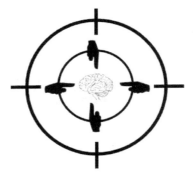

Stress and Working Memory

You are walking and enjoying a nice day at the park when suddenly, you find this unexpected reptile.

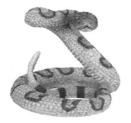

What would you do?
Probably jump or run.

When there is distress, working memory shuts down. When stress is present, the amygdala is activated since it is the fear sensor in the brain. The amygdala senses threat and coordinates with the motor cortex, sending the message, "You have to move!" Research has found that stress enhances executive motor control, which helps you have a quick reactive response and escape from the threat (Shields et al., 2016). When you see the snake, the amygdala is triggered, sending a message to the motor cortex "fight or flight." Your working memory is not necessary in fight-or-flight mode, so it is inhibited by your amygdala. At this point, the brain does not need to think of the situation but to move quickly, leaving the thinking for later. This is the natural safety process of your brain. You do not let your working memory figure out if this is a poisonous or a friendly snake. You just run. If working memory is involved in this process, by the time it brings previous information from your long-term memory file and analyzes whether this is a friendly snake or not, you would have already been bitten. So, no working memory in life-or-death situations.

Here is another scenario. You have a presentation prepared for your colleagues. You have studied very hard and know all the concepts. There is a small detail; you always feel nervous when you present in front of an audience. You are ready, and you see all the people in front of you, and suddenly, you forget your opening because your amygdala hits you with fear or stress, inhibiting your working memory. Your amygdala shuts down your prefrontal cortex because of the stress of talking in front of a group. When the amygdala is active, you cannot think. A meta-analysis showed that stress impairs working memory and cognitive flexibility, cognitive inhibition (Shields et al., 2016), and executive functions (Schoofs et al., 2009).

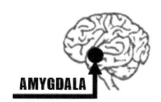

In the classroom, we want students to be ready with their working memory. If the students do not feel safe in the classroom, the amygdala is going to take over their working memory, and learning will not happen. We need students with functional working memory.

What are some situations in which students could feel threatened in the classroom?

Examples:

Layout of the classroom

Bullying

Disorganization

Placing the student on the hot seat

All of these situations put the amygdala to work and shut down working memory. The amygdala is the part of the brain responsible for emotions, survival, and emotional memory. The more fear you feel, the less you can think. In life-or-death situations, the brain shuts down the thinking process, and it has direct access to the cerebellum and motor cortex loop for movement purposes. The cerebellum receives information from the sensory systems and other parts of the brain and then sends a signal to the motor cortex to move. The cerebellum is responsible for balance, posture, coordination, speech, and voluntary movements. The cerebellum is a fundamental part of the brain since it represents ten percent of the brain but comprises fifty percent of the neurons.

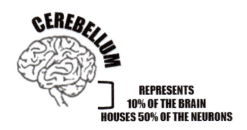

CEREBELLUM

REPRESENTS
10% OF THE BRAIN
HOUSES 50% OF THE NEURONS

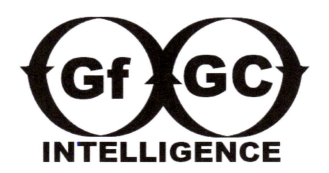

Fluid and Crystallized Intelligence

Solve the following.

Draw the next pattern in the sequence below.	Explain below why the American Flag has 50 stars and 13 stripes.
Answer:	Answer:

In 1963, Raymond Cattell described two intelligence categories, fluid and crystallized intelligence. Fluid intelligence (Gf) is the ability to solve new problems, use logic in a new situation, and identify patterns in sudden situations. When people figure out something in the moment and adapt to the situation, they just applied their fluid intelligence. When an individual figures out where to go on a map, he or she is using fluid intelligence. Studies have found strong relationships between working memory and fluid intelligence (Duncan et al., 2012; Ackerman et al., 2005; Kane and Engle, 2002; Kyllonen and Christal,1990).

Crystallized intelligence (Gc) is the ability to use learned knowledge and experience. Crystallized intelligence is used when you are taking a class or learning a new language. It is applied when people learn new vocabulary or the general rules of grammar. Crystallized intelligence accumulates over time, and it is information that we can access when necessary. In the first task, you experienced fluid intelligence when you had to solve a problem like the pattern. The second task is a crystallized intelligence activity in which you just bring back knowledge already learned.

Short term / Working memory (Gsm) is one of the five factors for IQ definition. The others are Crystallized intelligence (Gc), Fluid Intelligence (Gf), Visual Intelligence (Gv), Processing Speed (Gs).

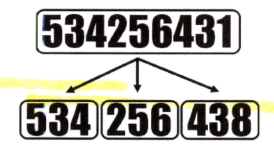

I Prefer It Chunked and Mixed

Let's try the next exercise.

Try to memorize the following colors.

Ready?

Close the book and say the colors.

Great! You just held three pieces of information.

Now, we will add a shape to the colors. Try to memorize them.

Ready?

Close the book and say the shapes and the colors.

Great! You just held six pieces of information.

We will add even more information. Try to memorize these. Ready?

Close the book and say the colors, shapes, and letters.

Super! You just held nine pieces of information, which is more than the average of seven.

Now let's manipulate the information in another way: Say the color, the shape, and the letter of the first item.

Now say the second item.

Now say the third item.

The process of retaining the information is easier when associations are involved. One of the ways working memory can manipulate the items is by saying the color, shape, and letter of the first item ✭ like in a column. The other way to manipulate the information is by saying the colors ○ ● ◉ in a row like shown in the figure.

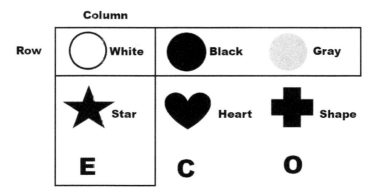

In addition, the information was chunked into sections, it was more digestible for the brain. First, you were given the colors, then another piece of information was added—the shapes—and finally, you were given the letters. Time was granted to process each chunk, which facilitated the retention. Imagine if you were given all the items at the same time. You would struggle to retain it all.

Probably, you made some associations that made the information easier to memorize. For example, some associate the black heart with feelings of being cold and the star with white like the star is shining, would make it easier to retain the items. If you know Spanish, you know that the word for heart is "corazón," which starts with "C." Another way to associate the items is by placing the letters together to form the word "ECO." Any resource available in the brain is helpful to hook new information to old information. The brain tries to associate something that is already known to something new and tries to make sense of the information for better cognitive retention. The more associations, the more neural pathways where the information could be stored.

One of the most famous examples of the power of associations is Dr. Ivan Pavlov's experiments. The test consisted of ringing a bell before feeding his dogs. The dogs came to associate the bell with food. When the bell rang, the dogs started to salivate even when there was no food involved. The sound of the bell constructed a pathway in the dog's brain announcing the food is coming—Yeah! Get ready!— and salivation began.

Let's try something different now with math. Try to solve the following problem in your mind.

12 X 9

There are different approaches to solving this problem, but let's analyze the one about chunking. Breaking down the number 12 into 10 and 2 would help to make the information more manageable. Now it would be easier to multiply 10 X 9 = 90 and hold that 90 in your working memory until you get the next computation. Then multiply 2 X 9 = 18, bringing back the 90 into the equation and add 90 + 18 = 108. This is working memory at its full function. Chunking the information helps to make mental calculations, but it depends on working memory capacity to maintain information on hold that would be used later in the task at hand. Mental math is a great way to develop and enhance working memory.

Researchers suggest that breaking down a cognitively demanding skill into smaller instructional units addresses the concern of overloading the cognitive capacity of students' working memory. It also helps students synthesize the information until it is mastered (Brophy and Good, 1986; Gersten et al., 2000; Hughes, 1998; Marchand-Martella et al., 2004; Rosenshine, 1997; Rosenshine and Stevens, 1986; Simmons et al., 1995; Swanson, 2001).

Students at a young age start using chunking techniques as a means to retain more information. The use of strategies is partly responsible for developmental increases in working memory. According to research, after age seven, children start to use rehearsal strategies (Gathercole, 1998; Gathercole et al., 1994; Gathercole and Hitch, 1993), including chunking (Ottern et al., 2007), and grouping (Bjorkland and Douglas, 1997).

Decomposing a word problem (high brain energy) cognitively demanding task

When working on word problems for the first time, chunk the problem by sentences. Provide the students only with the first sentence instead of the entire problem (chunking). Then ask them to read it and discuss it.

Lisa starts building the first layer of a rectangular prism using 34 cubes.

Something you would like to hear while you are monitoring throughout the classroom is that students are discussing who is the main character, vocabulary, and connection with real life. Also, students can draw or label for better understanding. Math word problems are written using topics that are familiar to students so they can make a connection with real events. In addition, math problems are stories like in reading. Provide questions and encourage discussion if necessary.

This is how the first sentence would look.

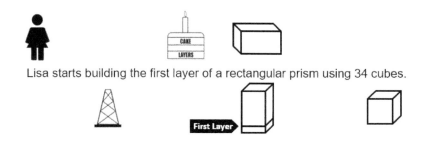

Lisa starts building the first layer of a rectangular prism using 34 cubes.

A word problem is like a story. It has a character, an action, and a problem to be solved.

Character – Lisa

What is Lisa doing? Trying to build a rectangular prism

Vocabulary – Cubes, layer, rectangular prism.

Now, reveal the second sentence and repeat the process.

Each cube has an edge length of 1 inch.

Once they have the second sentence, ask them to read it, and find vocabulary they may not understand. Then ask students to make a connection with the first sentence. With this process of decomposing problems, the thinking goes deeper, one sentence at the time, constructing meaning. In the beginning, it takes time, but in the long run, students will follow this process even later when they receive the full problem. We are also ensuring repetition because every time they receive another sentence, they have to go back and connect it with previous information.

Now reveal the next sentence and repeat the process.

The finished rectangular prism has 7 layers.

Repeat the discussion process and allow enough time to connect the three sentences.

Reveal the last sentence.

What is the rectangular prism's volume?

This activity should take around ten minutes and definitely could take as long as student discussions are focused. Here goes the first day of math problem-solving. Conversations and deep understanding are the benefits of this activity.

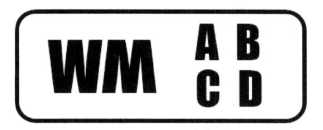

Working Memory and Reading

Read the following text.

> The brain is a voracious organ nourished by a sophisticated blood vessel system that consumes 20 percent of the energy of the body, equivalent to 10 to 23 watts, or enough to power a light bulb. This magnificent structure represents only 2 percent of the body mass, but its rapaciousness devours 10 times more energy than the rest of the body.

Cover the paragraph.

Retell as much information as you can to yourself or some else.

Your working memory helped you, retrieving from your long-term memory the specific connection with the text presented. Working memory associated new information with your background knowledge (anchor information) stored in your long-term memory. Students who make a connection based on their experience can retell more details of the text. Moreover, students with high working memory would retain more data from the text and can retell more details than those students with low working memory. Typically, children with poor working memory have trouble in these activities, disrupting the incremental learning process leading to poor academic growth (Gathercole et al., 2006). Children with reading disabilities have marked deficiencies on verbal working memory tasks in relation to average developing individuals (Seigel and Ryan, 1989; Swanson, 1999). Working memory is fundamental for complex cognitive processes such as spoken and written language, comprehension, mental arithmetic, reasoning, and problem-solving (Baddeley, 1988). Children's performance on measures of working memory serves as a useful predictor of several cognitive skills, including literacy (De Jong, 1998; Swanson and Berininger, 1995).

The retention and manipulation of certain sounds and letters in our brain is the job of working memory. The brain simultaneously activates different parts of the brain when reading a sentence. First, the brain must distinguish the visual structure of letters, order of letters, and segmentation. Then, the brain holds the sounds in working memory blending them into a recognizable word attaching meaning afterward. In a sentence, the reader must comprehend sentence syntax and language structure. Working memory helps hold several sentences while the process of comprehension is being handled. Some children might avoid reading due to poor working memory capacity. Poor working memory also translates into difficulty in retelling a story in their own words.

Studies have measured the average word span of most individuals is from five to ten words. Other studies showed that word span could be from five to as high as sixteen words (Baddeley et al., 1987). Other considerations include the length of words. When words are short, there is greater likelihood to have a better grasp. Word length plays a role in the recalling process. Words such as pay, jar, and net are more likely to be recalled since they are only three letters. Long words such as possibility, automatic, and transplant slow down the process of recalling and increase the probability of forgetting (Cowan et al., 1992; Dosher and Ma, 1998).

You can apply a working memory activity when reading aloud. After you read a page or a paragraph, ask students to retell as much as they can from the story. This is a practice students should do every time to enhance listening and verbal skills in the lower grade levels. By this practice, students would increase their working memory capacity. The previous activity is only recalling information, but we can include some manipulation after the retelling by asking for the character's feeling or the problem they need to solve in a fiction text.

Parents who read stories to their children are helping to expand their children's working memory. By rereading the same story over and over, they help children transfer the details of the story into their long-term memory. Reading new stories challenges the working memory and expands it. Asking questions about the text is a great opportunity to reinforce cognitive abilities.

For reading comprehension of the text, a student needs to read each sentence and hold it in their mind while also making sense of its meaning. The student would need to simultaneously process and store the information in the text over a short time. If the student is not able to retell much information from the text, this could be a red flag for most teachers about poor working memory capacity. Common failures of working memory during academic tasks are reflected in skipping letters or words, blending different words or sentences together, and losing track of sentences or numbers (Holmes et al., 2010).

So, what does this student's case suggest? Teachers, administrators, and parents need to become more aware of how cognitive functions like working memory affect the daily lives of students. It is estimated that eighty percent of children with poor working memory struggle with math, reading, or both (Gathercole and Alloway, 2008).

Anchor Information

Can you associate the shapes with numbers?

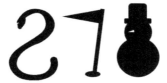

What number does it make?

_____   _____   _____

So what number did the shapes make? The answer:

278

What your brain did was to look at the shapes and match them to numbers. The old information, in this case, numbers, serves as anchor information connecting the new information, the shapes.

Anchor information is the material we rely on first to process another new piece of information. Let's say that a student has to multiply 6 X 6. He does not know the 6s multiplication facts, but he knows the 5s multiplication table in which 5 X 6 is 30. He adds another 6 to get the answer for 6 X 6 which is 36. The multiplication table of 5s served as an anchor to solve the problem at hand. Working memory serves as a retriever, soliciting anchor information from long-term memory to make sense of new information.

The same effect happens in reading when we do not know a word among others already known. We use context clues to figure it out. The words surrounding the unknown word serve as anchor information.

Example:

> The ocean was full of pesticides, herbicides, and **toxic** materials from irresponsible industrial disposal.

Using anchor information helps us know the meaning of an unknown word such as **toxic** in which we make an association with other words in the surroundings like pesticides, herbicides, and materials. The surrounding information helped to give us a clue as to what the word **toxic** means.

Example:

> The Sequoia National Park houses most of the **colossal** trees in the United States, specifically General Sherman, a giant sequoia tree.

Using anchor information helps us know the meaning of an unknown word such as **colossal**. We know that **colossal** refers to the trees, and giant tells us they are huge trees. The surrounding information helped to give a clue as to what **colossal** means. When the student reads this paragraph, the information has to be retained in working memory to make sense of the meaning of the message. In reading, you hold as much information as you can, and then you process the information to find meaning.

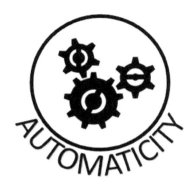

Automaticity: The Brain Liberator

Let's take some notes. Please grab your pencil and write the following sentence in the first rectangle.

Automaticity is the brain liberator.

Writing Hand

Now write it with your Non-Writing Hand

What difference did you notice in the process of writing with your writing hand and non-writing hand?

When you are using your writing hand, you accessed your cerebellum and motor cortex loop. You did not think about which hand would take the pencil; you just took the pencil because it is automatic. You never thought about how to position your pencil in your hand to start writing; you placed your pencil in your hand the way you always do (automatically).

Things change when you have to write with your non-writing hand. You use more effort. Working memory was activated in your non-writing hand, unless you practice writing with both hands and you have no problem, otherwise, some effort is required. By writing with your non-writing hand, you need to analyze the position of your fingers, taking the pencil, and imitating your writing hand. You have to remember or place more emphasis on how the letters look. What about speed? Can you write at the same speed as your writing hand? You require more effort. Working memory is active, helping you complete the task, and this means more energy is consumed because of the effort required by the chore.

Nowadays, repetition and memorization are considered outdated, but without it, we could not have a strong foundation for other challenging tasks. Our neural conductor needs raw material to put information together in a creative way. A good metaphor is when making a chair from scratch, we need the wood, raw material; without it, we cannot have a chair. In the case of problem-solving, such as 12x14, our raw material would be knowing the multiplication tables; without it, we could not solve the overall problem. It also applies to reading when providing raw material, such as learning the alphabet, to be able to read. What do we do with our kindergarten students when learning the alphabet? We make them repeat it every day until it is registered into their long-term memory. Once they know the alphabet, it becomes automatic, leaving the space and energy for the brain to deal with more cognitively challenging tasks. Younger children rely more on working memory due to having fewer automatic skills (Cowan, 2014). Once more, this is the reason reinforcing working memory is critical at a young age.

Let's do the next task:

When you see the circle, say its color.

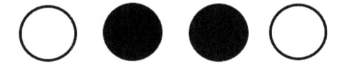

Easy, wasn't it?

Now when you see the circle say the opposite color of the circle. For example, when the circle is black, say white, and when it is white, say black.

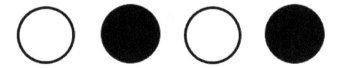

How was it?

In the first task, you said the colors automatically, so you did not use your working memory at all. In the second task, you needed to turn on your working memory to complete this task. It likely took you more time than the first task.

During automaticity, working memory is maintained out of the loop until an analysis of information is required. For experienced drivers, driving could be something automatic, and moreso if you follow the same route every day. It is like when you arrive at your destination without knowing the details of your driving. Let's say that you are driving in your regular mode and the same route, but there is an accident ahead, and you read in the electronic display by the highway, "Accident ahead on Judson Avenue." In this case, your working memory is required to evaluate the situation. What do you do? If you stay, you will be late for work. Should you get out of traffic? Should you find another route? You analyze the situation with the different components you observe and decide to find an alternative route. Working memory helps us to analyze and decide what to do with the information we have available and combine it with what is in long-term memory. Working memory searches the long-term memory files and finds what you need and combines it with what you are experiencing at the moment. Once this information is combined, decisions are made.

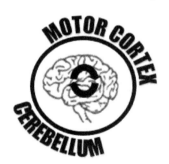

Automatization allows students to focus on the important, demanding tasks like comprehending a math problem. Let's say that you ask your students to solve 19 x 3, and in their minds, you know that the priority is to solve the problem, but the students do not know the multiplication tables. Not knowing the multiplication tables of 9 became a distractor from the priority, and this adds a step that could have been avoided if consistent practice on multiplication tables had been applied. A way to make it easier for student's working memory is to simplify things through automatization.

Research shows the brain does not require that much effort when you already know something. Knowing some information in automatic mode does not overload your working memory, saving the required expense of energy for critical tasks. Various studies had shown improvements when participants engage in short term memory task rehearsal (Gardiner et al., 1994; Rodriguez et al. (2000). Practice and repetition would greatly support the working memory system by preventing brain overload.

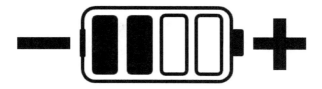

Cognitively Demanding
Tasks and Brain Energy

Let's work on the following task. Rephrase the question as an answer statement.

**How many miles does Addison need to run
to get to the finish line?**

Answer:

Addison needs to run _____ miles to get to the finish line.

What do you think? Would this task be a cognitively demanding task?

A cognitively demanding task requires more brain energy at the beginning until it is mastered. More regions in the brain are activated when there is a deep thought for the first time. Once the task is learned, fewer locations of the brain are needed and, of course, less energy spent.

The focus of the entire math word problem is the question. Students would be asked to make the question a statement. When students generate the answer statement, they would have a blank where the answer would be written. In this way, students could use some of the question structure to build the answer statement.

If it is a conversion problem, the student must be aware that it is asking for miles, not kilometers, or yards. The student is then be more focused on what to find. Also, with this process, students use part of the structure of the question to make it a statement.

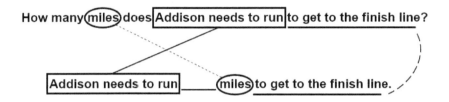

Some of the words from the question are used to structure the answer statement.

**Making decisions (high brain energy)
cognitively demanding task (focus)**

In some situations, students face the difficulty of what arithmetic operation to do in a word problem. This is where the cognitive load is more challenging because they need to decide what to do based on their understanding of the problem. Making decisions is where we want students to spend their energy and not on fundamental skills.

Automaticity (low brain energy)

Now, based on what the student needs to do, what activities or tasks do they need to be automatic? Going back to the metaphor of the chair in which your raw material is wood, without this good, strong wood, the chair would never be strong at all. The same happens with our students. Do they all have the raw material or foundations they need for a specific task?

Research shows that less energy is spent when a task is mastered, leaving brain energy for a challenging task. Automaticity help students use less brain energy on the task that is basic or foundational. Emphasis in practice would grant this automaticity for our students. So, our raw material becomes those foundational practices that are mastered with varied repetition.

Let's identify which activities should be already automatic tasks (foundational raw material) or cognitively demanding tasks.

Here are some math problems. Read them and write what task the student should already know and so should be automatic, and in the other column, write where the student should be spending their brain energy as a cognitively demanding task.

Aiden bought an old wooden collectible toy. He repaired and painted it, then sold it for $80.
- The cost of the old toy was $14.
- He spent 4 hours repairing with a cost of $2 per hour.
- He spent $6.50 in repair materials.

What was Aiden's profit after selling the old toy?

Automatic (Mastered foundations, our raw material)	Cognitively Demanding Task
• Align decimals • Addition with decimals • Multiplication • Vocabulary (cost and profit) • Using the question structure to formulate the answer statement	• Comprehension of the problem • Operation decisions (add, subtract, divide, or multiply) • Equation

Mrs. Martinez is putting a fence around the perimeter of her backyard.

- The perimeter of the backyard is 171 ft.
- Each section of the fence is 9 ft long and costs $8

How much money does Ms. Martinez spend putting the fence in her backyard?

Automatic (Mastered foundations, our raw material)	Cognitively Demanding Task

Maria and her two friends went to the rodeo and spent $84

- They spent $39 on food.
- They spent $24 on rides.
- They spent the rest on buying entrance tickets.

How much did they each pay for the entrance tickets?

Automatic (Mastered foundations, our raw material)	Cognitively Demanding Task

Miguel went to the store and bought light bulbs.
- He bought 12 light bulbs.
- Each of the light bulbs cost $3.49.
- He had a store discount of $2.95 off the total.

How much did Miguel pay for 12 light bulbs?

Automatic (Mastered foundations, our raw material)	Cognitively Demanding Task

Jesse is having an Italian party, so he went to the store and bought some food items.
- He bought 3 packets of pasta for $1.15 each.
- He bought 2 bottles of tomato sauce $2.35 each.
- He bought 1 container with parmesan cheese for $1.95.
- He used a store coupon for $1.85 off the total.

How much did Jesse spend on food items?

Automatic (Mastered foundations, our raw material)	Cognitively Demanding Task

Melissa and her two friends rode their scooters yesterday.

- Melissa rode her scooter for 9 kilometers.
- Brenda rode twice of Melissa's distance.
- Maria rode 3 kilometers less than Brenda.

What distance did Maria ride her scooter?

Automatic (Mastered foundations, our raw material)	Cognitively Demanding Task

Ask yourself, what does the student need for this assignment? What do they need to know to concentrate on the task at hand? Remember that you want to spend the working memory energy on the challenging task. You should have the raw material already mastered.

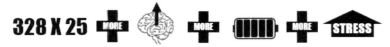

Cognitively demanding task + high concentration + high brain energy + high stress

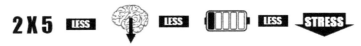

Automatic task − low concentration − low brain energy − less stress

A cognitively demanding task entails more effort and concentration by the brain. In addition, the brain spends more energy. At some point, the brain is going to get tired, and its efficiency will decrease. All of the tension would be concentrating on the cognitively demanding task provoking levels of stress to rise.

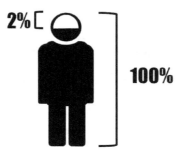

The brain represents only 2% of the body.

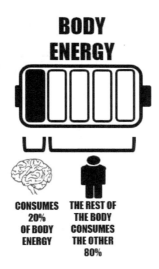

The brain consumes 20% of the energy.

Automaticity does not just apply to math. Here are some reading examples.

What automaticity is needed to understand this sentence?

1. Her head was spinning from the overload of information.

Automatic (Mastered foundations, our raw material)	Cognitively Demanding Task

2. After many tries, finally, opportunity knocked at his door.

Automatic (Mastered foundations, our raw material)	Cognitively Demanding Task

3. He is living his life in chains, being at school detention.

Automatic (Mastered foundations, our raw material)	Cognitively Demanding Task

This happens when we are teaching figurative language; students always find the literal meaning but not the hidden message.

1. Hyperbole – exaggeration to accentuate the point.
2. Personification – giving human characteristics to inanimate ideas, animals, or objects.
3. Symbolism – a word that has meaning but represents something else.

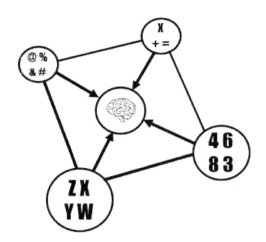

Brain Overload

If I asked you to learn all of this book by tomorrow, you would probably feel overwhelmed by the amount of information. The brain needs time to process and synthesize the information. Too much information in a short time causes a brain overload.

Let's answer this question first. On what day of the week do you introduce new information to your students? Let's say you have all this new content to introduce:

Reading: main idea
Writing: good conclusions
Math: fractions
Science: the water cycle
Social Studies: communities

Brain overload is caused by trying to absorb large quantities of information in a short time. Remember that the brain retains two to three pieces of information for a short time. The consistently varied practice would help this information to be stored into long-term memory. To engrave the information in the long-term memory, it has to be reviewed the first ten minutes after the introduction using the "ten and two rule," which is ten minutes of information for two minutes of reflection. After practicing the new information for the first time, review the information in the next 48 hours, and then again seven days after.

Overload of information certainly affects your working memory. Nowadays, we receive more information than we can process from different sources like television, cellphones, the internet, and emails. A solid working memory helps us select which information is relevant. A study found evidence that some stress effects could be present when there is a high working memory load (Oei et al., 2006). In this situation, when there is too much to process, working memory can shut down or crash, starting with the students with poor working memory.

Breaking down multiple steps into independent steps, repeating the information, and using instructional aids such as notes, reduces the working memory loads (Alloway, 2006; Gathercole and Alloway, 2004). Other supports for students include simplifying linguistic structures, reducing the length of sentences, and using familiar material.

Some suggestions to help students with poor working memory is managing the memory demands in the classroom. This can be possible if, for example, directions are chunked into a few steps. Also, repeating the information to the student over time. Making all the tools and manipulatives available for the student is a way to make content more comprehensible. Simplifying linguistic structures makes information more accessible to process for students with working memory challenges.

Routine is a working memory helper. When there is a routine already established, working memory is not at work. Asking students to do something different creates a demand for attention, erasing what was on their brain before and doing something in a different way, creating a brain overload. Remember to leave the brain load for the concepts or things you really want your students to learn.

When you have an organized environment in the classroom, it prevents a brain load by helping the students find the right materials at the right time for use. Some teachers use pictures for students to see where things go, preventing a brain load, and providing visual cues.

Some directions could be overwhelming for students creating a brain overload. Breaking down instructions is a brain support. Saying directions one at the time or in considerable chunks helps students. Wait until an instruction is carried out by students before going to the next step.

Some recommendations to help manage working memory are providing external aids, reducing processing difficulty, and preventing working memory overload.

Perspiration

Your brain is like any other muscle in the body—the more you exercise it, the better it performs. Training requires everyday perseverance to develop a habit and establish strong brain connections. Thomas Edison is often quoted as saying, "Genius is 1% inspiration and 99% perspiration." Without a doubt, inspiration is fundamental, but putting the hours into it makes the dream come true. How many times have we had a great idea but never followed up to make it a reality? That 99% perspiration is what makes things happen.

How much time spent on practice makes a huge difference? We probably do not know how much we need to practice, but research supports the quote from Jocko Willink: "The more you do it, the better you get." A study in 1990 by psychologist K. Anders Ericsson found that those who practiced ten thousand hours on the violin became elite violinists. The next group, with fewer hours of practice, just became good violinists. The third group, with the fewest hours of practice became music teachers and never become professionals. According to Guthrie, J. T. (2004), experts spend 500% more time practicing skills than beginners do. Research support that practice is the key to success.

Consistent practice allows you to make the task automatic and puts your working memory to rest. With persistent, varied practice, your brain does not think about the movements you need to do. The task at hand has been repeated so often that you do not have to make an effort to do it. This allows your brain and working memory to leave energy for tasks that are more cognitively demanding. When an assignment or task has been practiced so many times, working memory is not required, and it is pushed aside, leaving the cerebellum motor cortex loop to enter into play.

Sometimes students face the challenge of multistep problems, and they need to make decisions. In this process, the student is thinking about what to do—whether they need to add first and then multiply or add and then divide. Working memory is trying to keep all the pieces together and make a judgment with the information. Once the student decides to add first and then divide, if they had enough practice with these computations, then they automatically do the calculations allowing working memory to rest for a while preventing brain overload. But let say that they do not learn the multiplication tables well. They need to spend more energy trying to figure out what is three times five, stressing the brain and making this an added process. This is when practice makes a difference in brain overload. Effort makes a difference, and it comes with a toll to pay, which is spending more energy. The more effort, the more energy spent. The less effort, the less energy spent, and the less tired you will feel. Also, those students who have mastered many of the cognitively challenging tasks are not using their working memory and spend less brain energy. At the end of the day, you see students with more energy due to their improved working memory than those with poor working memory.

Students with poor working memory had two options when doing a task. One is to place a huge strain on working memory, trying to finish the task; obviously, brain energy would decrease. The other option is to shut down or quit the task early due to high cognitive demand. This might be the reason why some students do not finish their work. Various studies have shown there is improvement when participants engage in short-term memory task rehearsal (Broadly et al., 1994; Gardiner et al., 1994; Rodriguez, and Sadoski, 2000). Practice and repetition would greatly support the working memory brain system.

Energy

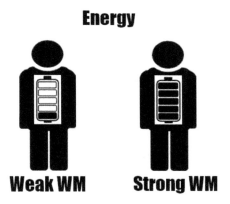

Weak WM   **Strong WM**

Research has shown that students with poor working memory may experience exhaustion at the end of the day due to brain overload.

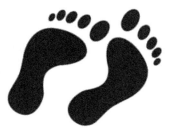

Fewer Steps, Fewer Mistakes

On the following exercise, if you want to have fun, you will need someone to read the next instructions to you. If you are by yourself, just read them and try to follow the instructions and act them out as quickly as you can.

Ready?

1. Act like a monkey
2 Rub your tummy
3. Clap three times
4. Say the vowels
5. Count backward from 6
6. Shake your hands in the air
7. Snap your fingers
8. Act like a chicken

Now keep the list hidden while you fill in the answers.

Recall the first instruction_____

Now the last one _____

What about the fourth one? _____

In a regular day, you ask students to follow instructions:

1-Get out your math journal.
2-Write your name in their next available page.
3-Show your thumbs up when ready.

You notice that several students just get their journals out. Hopefully, it's the math journal. Some students have their thumbs up because they are following others, but they never wrote their names in their journals. Some students took their journals out and stopped; they do not know what to do next. Observe your classroom when you give directions; you may have students with low working memory. Remember that this is a common behavior for students with poor working memory.

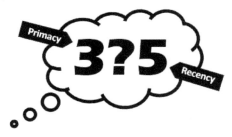

The brain tends to remember only the first and the last instruction. German psychologist Herman Ebbinghaus performed a series of studies on himself and found out that recalling instructions depends on the item's position on the series. He coined the term serial position effect, which is the tendency of recalling the first and the last items on the series effectively. When people are asked to recall the items, they recall the last one. This is called the recency effect. After the last item is mentioned, the people tend to name the first item more recurrently than the middle item. This is called the primacy effect.

Number of instructions able to be followed according to age.

Age	Instructions
5 to 6	2
7 to 9	3
10 to 12	4
13 to 15	5
16 to 39	6
40 to 49	5
50 to 59	4
60 to 69	3

The primacy effect and recency effect also apply to simple three-word instructions. When you tell your students, "Sharpen your pencil," they will get the last word pencil (recency effect) and sharpen (primacy effect).

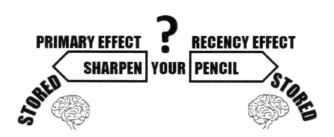

The words *sharpen* and *pencil* would have a privileged storage space in memory due to the primary and recency effect.

Primacy Effect	Instructions	Recency Effect
Sharpen	Sharpen your pencil	Pencil
Read	Read your book	Book
Bring	Bring your notebook	Notebook
Raise	Raise your hand	Hand

When giving instructions, provide only two to three instructions at the time, If possible, only two instructions. The brain mainly remembers the first and the last instruction, the first because you have all the students' attention, and they are waiting for what the teacher will say, and the last because it is the freshest information you received. The instructions in between will always be harder to remember due to a lack of relevance and focus.

Adults can manage three instructions, and they will implement them without trouble. But with students, it is more effective to use one or two instructions at a time. If you decide to give two instructions, you should not give more until those two directions are executed. Too many directions will confuse students, and some are not ready to follow them. Remember that 15% of your students have poor working memory, and you want 100% to follow the commands.

When giving instructions, follow these suggestions:

1. Establish eye contact – If you are talking to the entire classroom, sweep with your eyes from left to right. The intention is to have all the students' attention first.
2. Use clear voice and simple language.
3. Provide the one or two directions (Consider how many instructions your students can manage).

4. Wait until everything is executed before providing the next instruction.

5. Repeat the instruction if necessary or ask students to repeat the instruction to you.

6. Encourage your students to ask for clarification using a question, such as, would you please repeat the last part?

7. Supplement the instructions using body language and gestures.

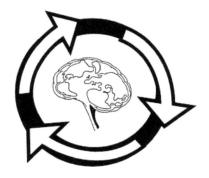

Long-term Memory:
The Final Journey

Think of a great vacation you had, like your honeymoon or a summer vacation to Hawaii.

Answer:_____

If you remember something, you are using your episodic memory where you stored important events or moments. Students use episodic memory when they are writing a narrative essay about their birthday, a graduation ceremony, or an exciting vacation. It all depends on how memorable the moment was to be able to retrieve as much information as needed.

Now, say the capital of Italy.

Answer:_____

If you said Rome, you are using your semantic memory, which encompasses facts or knowledge about the world. Students use this type of memory when you ask them what the capital of their state is, or who the mayor of their city is. Semantic memory also includes other types of information, considered general knowledge. Psychologist Endel Tulving in 1972, made the division of long-term memory into episodic memory and semantic memory. Information in long-term memory can be stored for long periods, even indefinitely, and can be accessed over more than a few seconds.

When you buttoned your shirt or tied your shoes, you used your implicit memory (also called "procedural memory"), which is unconscious and allowed you to do a task without thinking. Remember, when there is no effort, there is not much brain energy spent. With sufficient practice, individuals can transfer a challenging activity into an automatic, unconscious activity.

Please complete the next activity. Fill in the blanks to complete the words.

W_ND_WS   N_K_   K_EE_EX
    WA_M_RT   MCD_N_ _DS

When you see the word dioxide, you will be more likely to see the word again if you are presented with the simple letters di_x_de. This phenomenon is called priming. The term refers to the repeated exposure of a word or object. Priming makes concepts easier to recall when it is required. Sometimes the brain receives information in pieces, and the brain fills up the missing information with what makes sense to complete the message.

Explicit memory (also called "declarative memory") requires conscious thoughts such as recalling things from yesterday's lesson, like the order of operations during math or naming the landforms during science. Varied repetition provides a way to engrave information into long-term memory until it becomes less challenging to recall.

ANSWERS: WINDOWS, NIKE, KLEENEX, WALMART, MCDONALDS

Obviously, the intention is that students transfer all the information into long-term memory as quickly as possible; it could be done by expanding working memory. When information is repeated several times, students are able to retrieve the information with less effort.

Researchers estimate that repeated varied exposures of the information will be most effective if it appears over an extended period. Researchers stated that a word must be exposed as much as seventeen times so that students can learn it. When teachers are planning a lesson, targeted words should be identified to be repeated continuously in varied ways in context throughout the lesson.

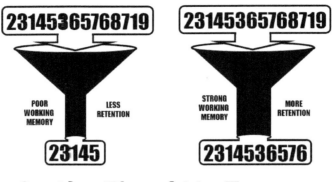

On the Tip of My Tongue

What is the word? I had it, but it is gone. This is what I said when I wanted to remember how to say snack in Spanish, I just had it in the tip of my tongue, but I forgot it. The trace of the memory disappeared. Later in the day, the word came back to me but not when I needed it, leaving me embarrassed in front of some friends. Tracing a memory depends on how strong the connections are in the retrieval process. When tracing a memory, there are small roads or highways in which retrieval is more accessible and some where it is not.

Our goal as teachers is that our students understand and remember what was taught and use it throughout their lives. How many times do we teach, and then the next day, students do not recall what was taught? Students sometimes look at us like they have never seen the information at all, while some of them give us some memory traces from the previous day.

German philosopher Hermann Ebbinghaus introduced the total time effect and the rule that the more time you invest in learning something, the better the information is stored. It is something like, "you get what you pay for." Reviewing notes immediately after the lesson is finished helps to retain eighty percent of the information. The review of the notes should happen in the following ten minutes after the lesson is over. Review again within forty-eight hours and before the week is over. Distributed and spaced practice is suggested instead of massing information in a single time.

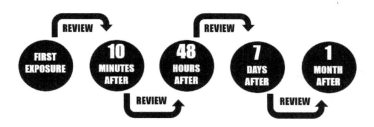

Review the information while it is fresh, typically ten minutes after the first exposure. Then review forty-eight hours after, seven days after, and one month after.

Distribution of practice effect confirms that spreading the information evenly over time is more effective than to mass the information in a single period. It is something like "little and often." The optimal way is by learning a little every day. Spaced presentation of the information enhances memory. When an item is taught for the first time, the sooner the item is tested, the better the possibility to be retained. This is why after you teach for the first time, you test the information learned in the ten minutes after it was taught.

The amount of time left after the first try would have some effect on relearning the information. When Hermann Ebbinghaus rehearsed his syllables for the second time one hour after, he had already forgotten some and spent half of the original time to relearn. When he rehearsed eight hours after, he has already forgotten some, and it took him two-thirds of the time to relearn. This shows the earlier you rehearse something, the less time it takes to relearn it. The longer you wait after the first try, the more time you need to relearn it. Rehearsal as quickly as possible while the information is still fresh is the key.

Time since the first exposure	Time needed to relearn
1 hour	½ of the time of the first exposure
8 hours	⅔ of the time of the first exposure

The length of time after the first exposure to information affects the time needed for the second review.

The quantity of the information to be learned affects rehearsal repetitions. When the information to be learned is short, the output of energy is low due to fewer repetitions. When the amount of information learned is considerable, the output of energy is higher, and there is a need for more repetitions.

The time needed for repetition decreased by everyday practice. It becomes easier, and less time is required to relearn it.

All of the information which is learned with effort is better retained. In contrast, the information easily learned fades faster, or put more succinctly, " easy come, easy go."

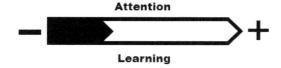

Making content interesting will attract student's attention and enhance retention. The amount of attention the student gives an interesting topic or item affects learning. On the other hand, if students are bored, this results in less attention, and less learning. More attention, more learning.

Here are some recommendations for how you can make the content more memorable.

If you want to ingrain learning, you need to be conscious of the following:

1. **Variation-** Repetition of information does not ensure retention by itself unless there is a variation of it. Repeating the same information over and over could be automatically ignored due to its tediousness. Presenting the information in different ways when reviewing is an effective way to aid retention.

   Example: If you taught the concept photosynthesis visually the first time, doing the same thing next time could fall because of repetition and provoke boredom for the students. On the contrary, if you review the concept photosynthesis by using body movement, there is repetition but a different presentation. When you try the previous strategies, you are building another pathway in the brain to retain the concept of photosynthesis, the first time with visuals and a second time with movements.

2. **Relevance-** A fundamental element for something to be learned and remembered is the meaning the learner gives to the information. If the information is not taught with attention to its use or relevance, the student will not be interested.

3. **Association-** Association between something already known and the new concept helps to hook meaning and retention.

4. **Redundancy-** This is a good predictor of the rated readability of material and its memorability. The more redundant and predictable a piece of prose, the easier it is to recall.

5. **Organization-** The organization of information helps to implant the information into the brain. The use of graphic organizers facilitates the retention of the information.

Example: Here is some information. Try to memorize it.

Chihuahua	Cats	Persian
Pug	Siamese	Poodle
	Dogs	Burmese

Now try to memorize it this way.

Dogs	Cats
Pug	Persian
Chihuahua	Siamese
Poodle	Burmese

For most people, the organized information is more memorable than the first list.

The way you present information is important. It affects retention and learning. Next time, use a graphic organizer to present the information to make it more useful and easier for the brain to absorb.

The first information is not organized but could be to be more brain-friendly by using a graphic organizer. Also, students could be taught to organize information by giving them different opportunities to categorize. Use different shapes and ask them to categorize according to the number of sides, vertexes, or faces.

6. **Connections**- Linking words by making a story leads to better retention of the information.

   Example: Try to link the next words into a story

   Pencil   bag   church   bench   book   table

   Now tell your story to your partner. This is another activity for students to find connections among words

7. **Imagery**- Visual imagery is a common technique when organizing material. If you have two words with no relationship at all, such as frog and stapler, you could create an image of the frog jumping from the stapler and making the noise when stapling. Certainly, an imaginative way to place these two words together into a single image allows the image to be even more memorable. If the imaginative visual in our brains is funny or unusual, the image gets trapped into the memory and can be recalled more easily. Moreover, if the two objects interact and have a kind of movement, making a movie or a scene, the possibilities of retention increase.

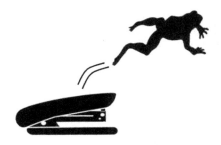

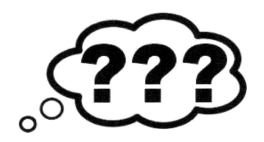

Forgetting

What did you do yesterday?
What did you do on this day last week?
What about this day a year ago?

You can probably recall what you did yesterday because it is most recent, and maybe last week because you had a memorable birthday party. What about one year ago on this day? We cannot remember unless it was a very important day in our lives; otherwise, it is difficult to recall. The student also would not remember what happened last year if it was not memorable. So, why do we forget? Some of the reasons could be because we simply cannot remember every detail of what we do; otherwise, we would have brain overload. With all the influx of information, the brain has learned to be selective. It is wise to concentrate on what we think is important, such as the date of a marriage proposal or the last birthday party. Do you remember what you were wearing at your last birthday party? You probably remember the event and the fun, but you were likely not paying attention to what you were wearing. If you do remember, perhaps it's because you took great effort in deciding what to wear, or maybe you spilled ketchup on your bright white shirt that day. What I mean is, something happened out of the ordinary that makes you remember this detail.

According to Ebbinghaus's studies on himself, the rate we forget is rapid at the beginning but slows down as time goes on. Those older memories are more resistant to decay than the recent ones.

There are two theories of forgetting. One is that memories just fade, and the other is that memories are disrupted by recent learning. This is why continuous practice is needed because the longer the delay in reviewing, the greater the forgetting. Also, the less interference in the material learned, the better the retention. Studies have found that students who study at night and then go to sleep, retain more material than those who study in the morning, and then have other activities during the day. The process of consolidation of memory operates during sleeping. This is why retention is better.

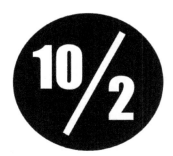

To have better results with retention, apply the 10/2 rule. It means that for every ten minutes of the teacher talking, allow two minutes of student reflection of the information.

Retroactive interference is an effect that happens when old information is forgotten due to the input of new information. It also depends on how weak is the old information. If this is the case, new strong information will weaken the old one even more, making it an interference.

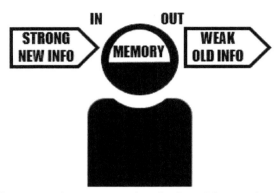

One of the examples I use is that before I learned English, I mispronounced the word island. Since Spanish is so phonetic, I used to pronounce the "s" in the word island, which makes it sound like Iceland. I had a hard time trying to eliminate this bad habit, so I have a retroactive interference. Once I received the new strong information that the "s" was silent, I corrected my old information and pronounced the word correctly.

Which one of these two words do you think would stay in your memory?

caution   sailor

If you say caution is a stronger word than sailor, perhaps you have an image of the word caution as a warning sign, and this has a greater imprint in your brain. Others might say sailor because they have a strong association with it. There are no wrong or right answers. It all depends on your experiences.

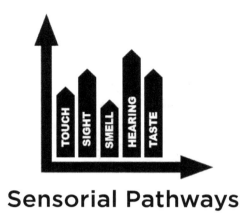

Sensorial Pathways

Imagine that you only have one sense to choose, which one will you keep? Circle your choice.

Now imagine that you have to get rid of one of the senses, Which one would you give away? Circle your choice.

Most of the people chose vision as the number one preference, and indeed vision is the most powerful sense, but which one is the most used in our classrooms? 91.2% of students' time is spent in whole group instruction (Pianta, R. et al., 2007). We structure our teaching as if students' most developed sense is hearing. Involve the senses in the classroom more often, especially vision, since it is the most powerful sense of all. After all, an image is worth a thousand words.

Why are some events more memorable than others? Most of it is due to the use of senses. How can we remember a specific aroma? And how do we relate it with an event in our lives? In my case, every time I smell new plastic, I remember my old toys. The sense of smell is powerful because it is close to the hippocampus, the place for long-term memories.

It is not that memory chooses what would be engraved or not; rather, it all depends on how we receive the information and how aware we are. Let's say that someone pinches you in the arm. Would you remember? Would you remember so you can pinch back? The association of the pinch with the face of the one who did it triggers your memory to try to find vengeance. Physical feelings like the pinch in your arm, the pain, got stored in your memory. So, it depends on the source of information and how you received that information. This combination would make a good memory stored for a longer time.

It is also true that words hurt even though they are not bad words. If one of your best friends suddenly tells you that she/he is not your friend anymore, you will remember those words because it made an impression, and it will be stored as the day I lost my friend.

Some memories have been stored since childhood, both good or bad memories, and they can be retrieved at any time as needed. There are other memories that we can't recall even if they happened yesterday or an hour ago. Even if you brushed your teeth two hours ago, you sometimes wonder if you did.

A great example of how the brain uses different pathways is the experiment of scientist Karl Lashley who trained rats to go through a maze for a food reward. He removed parts of the cerebral cortex to see if the rats were able to remember the maze, and they still did. He removed almost 90% of the rats' cerebral cortex, and they were still able to run the maze. He wrongly concluded that only 10% of the brain was needed for memory. What he actually discovered is that the brain uses different pathways to engrave a memory through their different senses. The motivation of the rats awakens all their senses to get the goal—food—engraving the information about the maze in different parts of the brain.

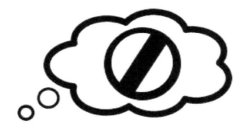

Inhibiting Distractions

For the next activity, time yourself.

Say the color of each one of the words. Ready?

WHITE   GRAY   **BLACK**

GRAY   **BLACK**   WHITE

BLACK   WHITE   GRAY

Time: _____

We will go again

Time yourself on the next activity as well.

Say the color of each one of the words. Ready?

WHITE   **GRAY**   BLACK

BLACK   GRAY   WHITE

WHITE   GRAY   **BLACK**

Time: _____

Was there a difference in your times?

Inhibition in this activity is the ability to suppress the automatic dominant response. In 1935, John Ridley Stroop published the effect, which is a demonstration of the reaction time of a task. The Stroop test is a great instrument to test whether individuals can inhibit distractors and focus on the assigned task. Working memory is also characterized by inhibiting distractors. Research states that people with great working memory can better focus and inhibit distractors. Dempster and Corkhill (1999) stated that inhibition when controlling for working memory is related to attainment and supports general academic learning. Inhibiting information also comes into play in language; researchers have found that reading a paragraph requires inhibiting the unnecessary information (Gernsbacher, 1993). Another approach to help students with poor working memory is to reduce distractions, so the inhibitory process is kept at a minimum or not used at all (Dempster and Crokhill, 1999).

Here are other tasks.

In the next activity, you will be timing yourself as well.

Read the words inside the animals. Ready?

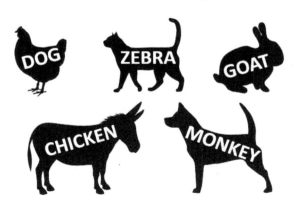

Time_____ (reading the words)

Now, you will see the graphics again, but this time, you will say the animal silhouette. Ready?

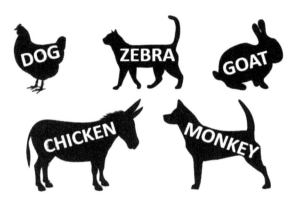

Time _____ (saying the animal of the picture)

Which attempt was more successful?

In this task, you have to be able to concentrate either on the visual or the word, according to the instructions. The information is overlapped to have interference. In which of the task, did you have more trouble? More visual people would be more successful with the images. Others who are more verbal would see the words more accessible than the pictures. The difference could be only fractions of a second between the two tasks, and you may not have noticed it.

Here is another example, but this time we will include some working memory and distractors to work with.

Look at and memorize the letters for the next task.

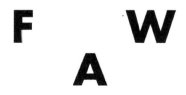

Cover the letters.

Can you identify any of the letters from the previous task?

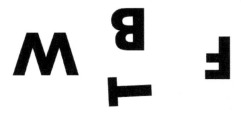

Which letters are those? _____

Which letters are distractors? _____

In this activity, you have to memorize the letters in the first task. Then you have to identify the letters from the previous task. Those letters were F and W, B, and T are distractors. Another distractor is the rotation of the letters, which makes it more difficult to identify. Also, there is a manipulation of the letters with the rotation. Even if the W looks like an M, you know that is W because all of the letters were moved.

One more activity to inhibit information.

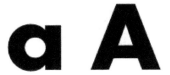

When you see the lowercase a, sit down and clap once. When you see the uppercase A, stand up and clap twice. Ready?

a A a A a A

a a A A a A

In this next task, you will do the same things. When you see a lowercase letter, it means you sit down and clap once. An uppercase letter means you stand up and clap twice. In addition, if the letters are white, follow these instructions. But if the letters are black, follow the opposite instructions. Let's practice.

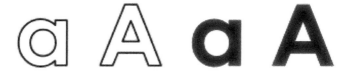

Let's do a longer sequence.

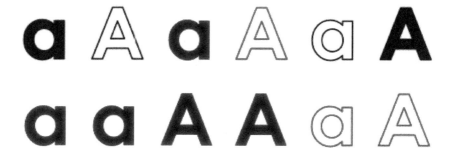

How did it go?

Since the brain relies more on conscious thinking, there is a delay. We have told our brains at the beginning that black means following the same rules but now in the second trial black means doing the opposite which delays the process. At the beginning, the colors have a set meaning in our brains, and resetting them with different meanings afterwards makes it more challenging.

PART II
THE HOW

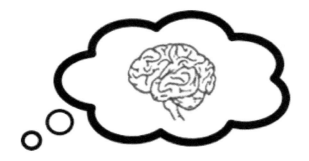

Training Working Memory

Exposing students to working memory activities will improve some proven cognitive abilities. There is a rapidly growing number of studies demonstrating that training in working memory capacity can yield improvements in a range of important cognitive skills (Chein and Morrison, 2010). Furthermore, training greatly enhances a student's ability. Children as young as preschool age have benefited from training their cognitive abilities (Thorell et al., 2008).

Students that had trained their working memory through computerized games had improved their math and reading scores. Working memory training includes spatial skills, letters and words, and mathematical operations. An advantage of training working memory is that students pay better attention because it allows them to inhibit distractions in their surroundings and focus on the information to be retained. When students work on a working memory task, they expand their capacity to absorb more information and understanding. Another benefit of continuing practicing working memory tasks is that it has transfer advantages into better scores.

Beyond awareness of how different cognitive functions, like working memory, can impact behavioral and academic performance, there is a feeling that the student has poor working memory and will suffer academically. But what should we do? A gradual working memory training would support this gap in academics. Researchers found that if they used tasks initially developed to test working memory and instead made them progressively more difficult within a training program that this could improve working memory capacity (Klingberg et al., 2002). This was an important discovery because previously working memory was believed to be a fixed cognitive capacity. Working memory training helped students gain substantial improvements in mathematical ability (Holmes et al., (2009).

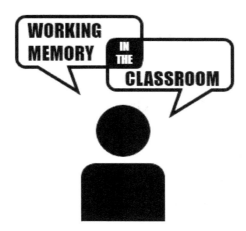

Working Memory Activities for the Classroom

There is some computerized working memory training out there, but I wanted to provide a simple way to apply more practice into the classroom. The exercises in this book are focused on students and will help them use their working memory as well as learning the content at the same time. Students can take advantage of the working memory practice and content getting a double benefit. With practice and dedication, you can expand students' memory to levels you cannot imagine. Training and exposure of students to working memory activities would greatly add cognitive advantages.

In addition, trained teachers can combine some content with working memory activities as a warm-up at the beginning of the lesson. One of the fundamentals of working memory is that you can make almost any activity into a working memory task following the protocol provided in this book. Think about what is important in the lesson, and focus the energy to create a working memory task using this specific content information. Also, there is a lesson plan template included for you to use to start creating your own working memory activities.

WHEN TO USE WORKING MEMORY ACTIVITIES

- As an everyday warm-up before beginning the lesson.
- As an extracurricular activity after school.
- During ancillary time or specials time
- After school enrichment classes
- Enrichment summer school
- During stations or centers
- When students are finished with their assignment
- As an extension of content
- As a transition activity for a few minutes
- To develop background knowledge as an introduction of a lesson
- Just for fun!

HOW DO WE DO IT?

There are many ways to do it:

- Whole group, projecting the activity or writing the information on the whiteboard.
- Individually (providing a sentence stem to help the oral language)
- Partners during stations
- Students who finish their assignment early as a way to improve their mental agility
- Make a desk station, where students can take a working memory assignment and review when they finish their content assignment early.

Activities are short and can develop attention patterns where they are needed.

These working memory activities could be accompanied by sentence starters to facilitate oral proficiency and discussion.

USE THE PROTOCOL FOR WORKING MEMORY ACTIVITIES

Follow the protocol for working memory.

1. Ask students to be attentive and quiet.
2. Show the information to be memorized for a few seconds (5 to 10 seconds), then take it away.
3. Ask for recall of the information.
4. Ask the manipulation questions provided.

Consider whether the students should answer individually orally, or with a partner taking turns. Make sure to monitor around the classroom so everyone participates. Also, make sure to pair students according to their oral skills. You can ask students to respond in complete sentences or use a sentence starter to support language development.

Remember to do this mentally, no paper allowed. Their scratch paper is in their brain. Let's expand it!

Let's apply working memory content to a classroom situation.

The next activity requires students to know the fact families.

Say or show students the two numbers below for about 5 seconds.

For example:

5   4

Recall: Ask students to recall the two numbers first. Answer: 5 and 4.

Manipulation: Ask students to say the fact family for multiplication and division that includes the numbers 5 and 4.

$$5 \times 4 = 20$$
$$4 \times 5 = 20$$
$$20 \div 4 = 5$$
$$20 \div 5 = 4$$

Students receive the stimuli through the auditory or visual sense (5 and 4). Then, this information is stored temporarily in working memory so that they can recall the two numbers. In the manipulation process, a signal is sent to long-term memory to recall the multiplication tables for 5s. Once the student has this information, working memory would make the calculation giving an output. Now, the brain and mouth should work together to articulate an oral response.

Here is another example.

The next activity requires students to know the alphabet.

Say or show students two letters for about 5 seconds.

For example:

F   A

Recall: Ask students to recall the two letters first. Answer F and A.

Manipulation: Ask students to say the letters in alphabetical order.

A   F

Students receive the stimuli through the auditory or visual sense (A and F). Then, this information is stored temporarily in working memory so that they can recall the two letters. In the manipulation process, a signal is sent to long-term memory to recall alphabetical order. Once the student has this information, working memory would make the categorization giving an output. Now, the brain and mouth should work together to articulate an oral response.

Process of exposure to working memory activities.

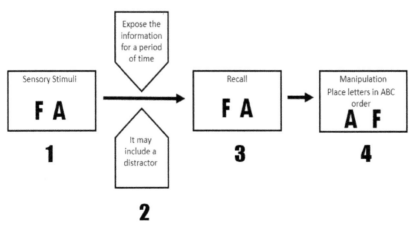

1. Senses detect stimuli
2. Visual exposure of the stimuli for a short time (it may include a distractor)
3. Recall of the information
4. Manipulation of the information

Working BRAIMemory

50+

Interactive Working Memory
Content Based Activities

1–Place Value

Say–I am going to show you a number. Be attentive and memorize them.

Challenge 1

547

Ask the following questions.

Recall
Say the numbers – 547.

Manipulation
What position does the number 4 occupy? The number 4 occupies the tens position.

What position does the number ___ occupy? The number ___ occupies the _____ position.

More examples

Challenge 2	Challenge 3
672	486

Challenge 4	Challenge 5
908	579

2–Least or Greater Than

Say–I am going to show you some numbers. Be attentive and memorize them.

13   26

Ask the following questions.

Recall

Say the numbers – 13 and 26.

Manipulation

Which number is the greatest? _____ is greater than _____.

Which number is the least? _____ is less than _____.

What position defines which is bigger? The _____ position defines which is the bigger number.

More examples

Challenge 2		Challenge 3	
23	46	43	62
Challenge 4		Challenge 5	
53	19	21	26

3–Two Shapes Overlapping

Say–I am going to show you some shapes. Be attentive and memorize them.

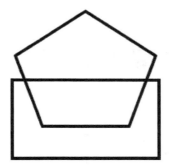

Ask the following questions.

Recall

Say the shapes in the figure – Pentagon and rectangle.

Manipulation

Say the shapes from top to bottom. Pentagon, rectangle.

Say the shapes from bottom to top. Rectangle, pentagon.

More examples

4–Three Shapes Overlapping

Say–I am going to show you some shapes. Be attentive and memorize them.

Challenge 1

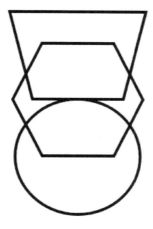

Ask the following questions.

Recall
Say the shapes in the figure – Trapezoid, hexagon, and circle.

Manipulation
Say the shapes from top to bottom. Trapezoid, hexagon, and circle.

Say the shapes from bottom to top. Circle, hexagon, and trapezoid.

Which shape is in the middle? Hexagon.

More examples

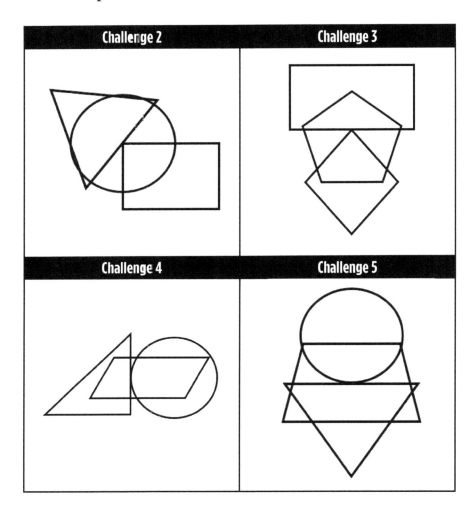

5–Verbs

Say–I am going to show you some verbs. Be attentive and memorize them.

JUMP
READ
SIT DOWN

Ask the following questions.

Recall
Say all the verbs – Jump, read, and sit down.

Manipulation
What verbs help you to learn?

The verbs that help me learn are _____.

What verbs help you exercise?

The verbs that help me exercise are _____.

What verbs help you relax?

The verbs that help me relax are _____.

More examples

Challenge 2	Challenge 3
WRITE SLEEP ROW	CLIMB STUDY LAY DOWN
Challenge 4	Challenge 5
RUN LISTEN RECLINE	TALK LEAN SWIM

6-Antonyms

Say – I am going to show you some words. Be attentive and memorize them.

Challenge 1

CLOSE
DOOR
OPEN

Ask the following questions.

Recall
Say the words – Close, door, and open.

Manipulation
Say the words that are antonyms. Close and open

Make a connection among the words – you can open and close a door.

More examples

Challenge 2	Challenge 3
APART FAMILY TOGETHER	SIT DOWN CHAIR STAND UP
Challenge 4	Challenge 5
BEST HOMEWORK WORST	BLAME DIPLOMA PRAISE

7-Synonyms

Say – I am going to show you some words. Be attentive and memorize them.

Challenge 1

ASK
QUESTION
INQUIRE

Ask the following questions.

Recall
Say the words – Ask, question, and inquire.

Manipulation
Say the words that are synonyms – Ask and inquire.

More examples

Challenge 2	Challenge 3
DIFFICULT HOMEWORK HARD	GATHER INFORMATION COLLECT

Challenge 4	Challenge 5
VALUE GRADE WORTH	RECOGNITION DIPLOMA PRAISE

8–Rounding to the Nearest Ten

Say- I am going to show you a number. Be attentive and memorize them.

Challenge 1

24

Ask the following questions.

Recall
Say the number - 24

Manipulation
Round the number to the nearest ten - 20

More examples

Challenge 2	Challenge 3
85	65
Challenge 4	**Challenge 5**
51	95

9-Rounding to the Nearest Ten and Hundred

Say–I am going to show you a number. Be attentive and memorize them.

51

Ask the following questions.

Recall

Say the number - 51

Manipulation

Round the numbers to the nearest ten. 50

Round the number to the nearest hundred. 100

More examples

Challenge 2	Challenge 3
84	136
Challenge 4	**Challenge 5**
249	396

10-Estimating the Number

Say–I am going to show you some numbers. Be attentive and memorize them.

Challenge 1

45   32

Ask the following questions.

Recall

Say the numbers – 45 and 32

Manipulation

Round the numbers to the nearest ten. 50 and 30.

Add the two rounded numbers. The answer is 80.

More examples

Challenge 2		Challenge 3	
35	49	61	23

Challenge 4		Challenge 5	
19	12	43	82

11-Dots

Say–I am going to show you an illustration for a few seconds. Be attentive and memorize it.

Challenge 1

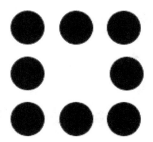

Remove the illustration.

Ask the following questions.

Recall

Say the number of dots - 8 dots.

Manipulation

How many dots are there if you complete the array? 9 dots.

How many dots go in the middle? 1 dot.

More examples

12-Double the Number

Say—I am going to show you some numbers. Be attentive and memorize them.

Challenge 1

15   25

Ask the following questions.

Recall
Say the numbers — 15 and 25

Manipulation
Double the numbers - 30 and 50

Add the doubled numbers - 80

More examples

Challenge 2		Challenge 3	
12	25	25	22
Challenge 4		**Challenge 5**	
20	35	40	20

13–Half the Number

Say–I am going to show you some numbers. Be attentive and memorize them.

Challenge 1

8   12

Ask the following questions.

Recall
Say the numbers – 8 and 12

Manipulation
Half the numbers - 4 and 6

Add the halved numbers - 10

More examples

Challenge 2		Challenge 3	
12	24	10	22
Challenge 4		**Challenge 5**	
14	20	16	24

14-Double the First Number and Half the Second

Say–I am going to show you some numbers. Be attentive and memorize them.

5   16

Ask the following questions.

Recall
Say the numbers – 5 and 16

Manipulation
Double the first number - 5 = 10

Half the second number -16 = 8

Add the results - 18

Multiply the results - 10 X 8 = 80

More examples

Challenge 2	Challenge 3
8 4	4 14
Challenge 4	**Challenge 5**
5 18	3 12

15–Arrays

Say–I am going to show you some colored dots. Be attentive and memorize them.

Challenge 1

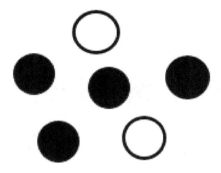

Ask the following questions.

Recall

Say the number of dots - 6

Manipulation

How many are white? 2

How many are black? 4

Mention the different arrays you can make with these dots. 2x3, 3x2,1x6, and 6x1

More examples

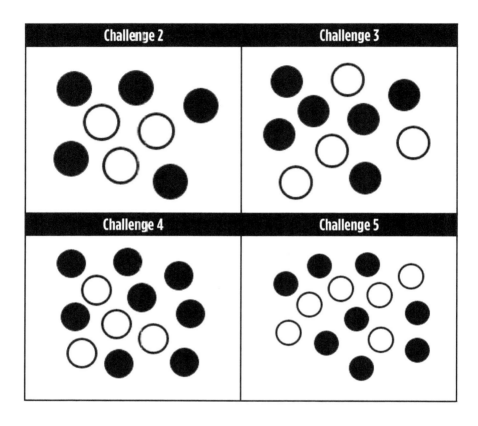

16-Whole and Part Model (Adding)

Say–I am going to show you a diagram. Be attentive and memorize it.

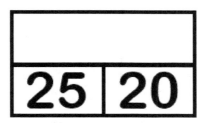

Ask the following questions.

Recall

Say the numbers - 25 and 20

Manipulation

Complete the missing part. Add the two numbers - 45

More examples

Challenge 2	Challenge 3
15	25	40	35

Challenge 4	Challenge 5
25	35	45	35

17-Whole and Part Model (Subtracting)

Say–I am going to show you a diagram. Be attentive and memorize it.

Challenge 1

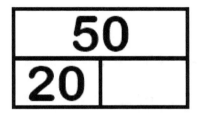

Ask the following questions.

Recall

Say the numbers - 50 and 20

Manipulation

Complete the missing part. Subtract the two numbers - 30

More examples

Challenge 2	Challenge 3
40	70
10	30

Challenge 4	Challenge 5
60	80
20	30

18–Subtracting Numbers

Say–I am going to show you some numbers. Be attentive and memorize them.

12   23

Ask the following questions.

Recall

Say the numbers – 12 and 23

Manipulation

Subtract the numbers - 11

More examples

Challenge 2		Challenge 3	
32	12	43	13
Challenge 4		**Challenge 5**	
12	52	62	12

19-Add and Double the Number

Say–I am going to show you some numbers. Be attentive and memorize them.

Challenge 1

14   7

Ask the following questions.

Recall

Say the numbers – 14 and 7

Manipulation

Add the numbers - 21

Double the result - 42

More examples

Challenge 2		Challenge 3	
12	13	22	12
Challenge 4		**Challenge 5**	
33	13	42	13

20-Ten Frames

Say–I am going to show you a diagram. Be attentive and memorize it.

Challenge 1

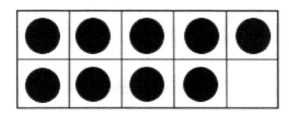

Ask the following questions.

Recall

Say how many dots are there–9

Manipulation

How many empty boxes? 1

More examples

21-Adding Coins

Say–I am going to show you some coins. Be attentive and memorize them.

Challenge 1

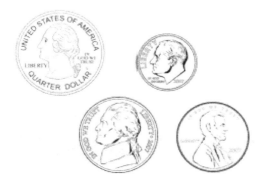

Ask the following questions.

Recall

Say the coins – Quarter, dime, nickel, and penny

Manipulation

How much money is there? 41 cents

More examples

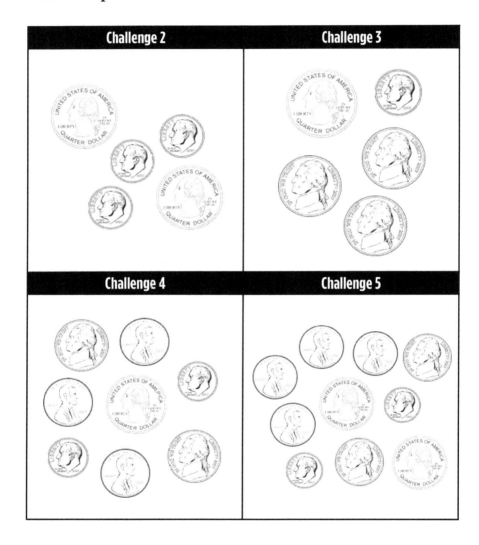

22–2D Shapes

Say–I am going to show you some 2D shapes. Be attentive and memorize them.

Challenge 1

Ask the following questions.

Recall
Name the images – square and pentagon

Manipulation
Describe the shapes.

How many vertexes? Square 4, pentagon 5

How many sides? Square 4, pentagon 5

How are they similar? Both are shapes

How are they different? Have different numbers of vertexes and sides

More examples

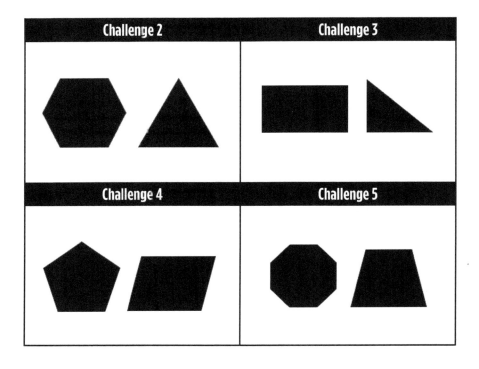

23-3D Shapes

Say–I am going to show you some 3D shapes. Be attentive and memorize them.

Challenge 1

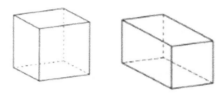

Ask the following questions.

Recall

Say the images – cube and rectangular prism

Manipulation

How many vertexes? The cube has 8 vertexes, and the rectangular prism has 8 vertexes

How many faces? The cube has 6 faces, and the rectangular prism has 6 faces

How many edges? The cube has 8 edges, and the rectangular prism has 8 edges

How are they similar? Both are 3D shapes and have the same number of vertexes, faces, and edges

How are they different? The cube has 6 faces, all the same size, but the rectangular prism's faces are different sizes.

More examples

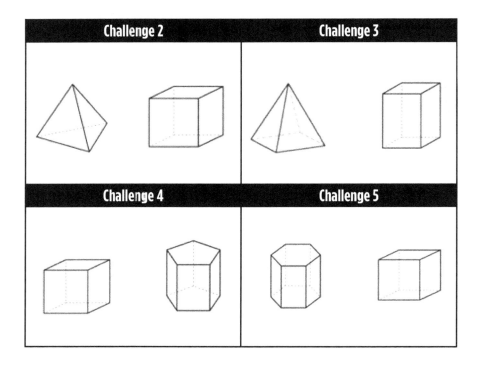

24–Constructing a 3D Shape

Say–I am going to show you some 2D shapes. Be attentive and memorize them.

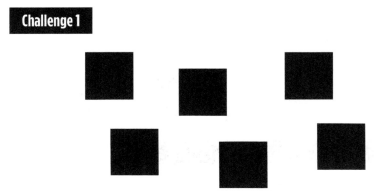

Ask the following questions.

Recall

How many shapes? 6 shapes

What shapes did you see? 6 squares

Manipulation

What 3D shape can you create placing all shapes together? You can create a cube.

175

More examples

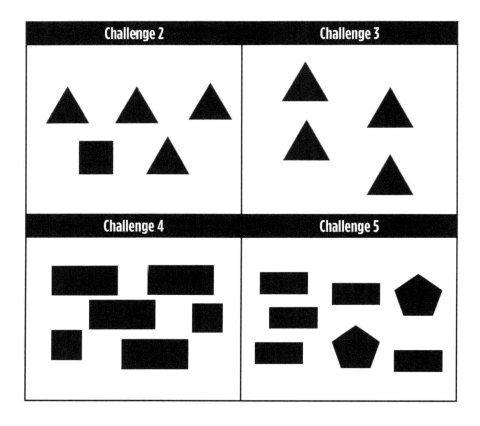

25-Multiple Operations

Say–I am going to show you some numbers. Be attentive and memorize them.

2   6

Ask the following questions.

Recall
Say the numbers – 2 and 6

Manipulation
Add the numbers - 8

Subtract the numbers - 4

Multiply the numbers - 12

Divide the numbers - 3

More examples

Challenge 2	Challenge 3
9 3	4 8
Challenge 4	**Challenge 5**
15 3	12 4

26-Converting Improper Fractions into Mixed Fractions

Say–I am going to show you a fraction. Be attentive and memorize it.

Challenge 1

$$\frac{3}{2}$$

Ask the following questions.

Recall

Say the improper fraction – Three halves

Manipulation

Make the mixed fraction: $1\frac{1}{2}$

More examples

Challenge 2	Challenge 3
$\dfrac{5}{4}$	$\dfrac{10}{3}$
Challenge 4	**Challenge 5**
$\dfrac{13}{4}$	$\dfrac{15}{4}$

27–Converting Mixed Fractions into Improper Fractions

Say–I am going to show you some numbers. Be attentive and memorize them.

$$1\frac{1}{2}$$

Ask the following questions.

Recall

Say the mixed fraction – one and one-half

Manipulation

Make the improper fraction: $\dfrac{3}{2}$

More examples

Challenge 2	Challenge 3
$1\dfrac{1}{4}$	$3\dfrac{1}{3}$
Challenge 4	Challenge 5
$3\dfrac{1}{4}$	$3\dfrac{3}{4}$

28-Family Facts

Say–I am going to show you some numbers. Be attentive and memorize them.

2   6

Ask the following questions.

Recall

Say the numbers – 2 and 6

Manipulation

Say the family facts.

$2\times6=12$

$6\times2=12$

$12\div6=2$

$12\div2=6$

More examples

Challenge 2	Challenge 3
4 5	3 4
Challenge 4	**Challenge 5**
5 9	6 8

29-Spelling Words

Say–I am going to show you some letters. Be attentive and memorize them.

net

Ask the following questions.

Recall

Spell the word – n, e, and t

Manipulation

Spell the letters from right to left – t, e, and n

More examples

Challenge 2	Challenge 3
tan	shoe

Challenge 4	Challenge 5
Note	idea

30–Creating Words

Say–I am going to show you some letters. Be attentive and memorize them.

r   e   a

Ask the following questions.

Recall
Recall the letters – r, e, and a

Manipulation
Say the letters from right to left – a, e, and r

Create words with the letters. are, ear, and era

More examples

Challenge 2			Challenge 3		
i	t	p	t	c	a
Challenge 4			**Challenge 5**		
n	a	t	m	a	r

Challenge 1: Tip, pit

Challenge 2: Act, cat

Challenge 3: Tan, ant

Challenge 4: Arm, ram

31–Visuospatial Practice 1

Say–I am going to show you an illustration. Be attentive and memorize it.

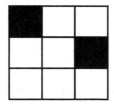

Show the next illustration.

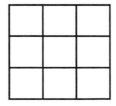

Ask the following question while you show the empty illustration.

Recall
Where were the shaded squares located?

Manipulation
Rotate the shape one time to the right and mention the shaded squares.

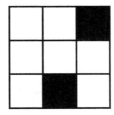

Note: Students can point at where the shaded squares when talking to another student.

More examples

32-Visuospatial Practice 2

Say–I am going to show you an illustration. Be attentive and memorize it.

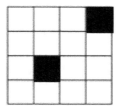

Show the next illustration.

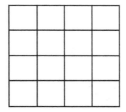

Ask the following question while you show the empty illustration.

Recall

Where were the shaded squares located?

Manipulation

Rotate the shape one time to the right and mention the shaded squares.

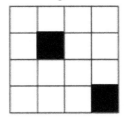

Note: Students can point at where the shaded squares when talking to another student.

More examples

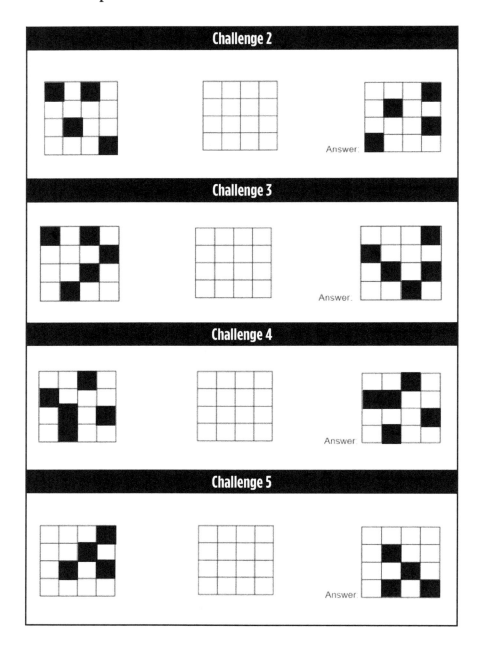

33–Fractions

Say–I am going to show you a figure. Be attentive and memorize it.

Challenge 1

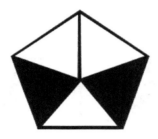

Ask the following questions.

Recall

How many parts? 5 parts

Manipulation

What is the fraction of the shaded part? Two-fifths

What is the fraction of the not shaded part? Three-fifths

More examples

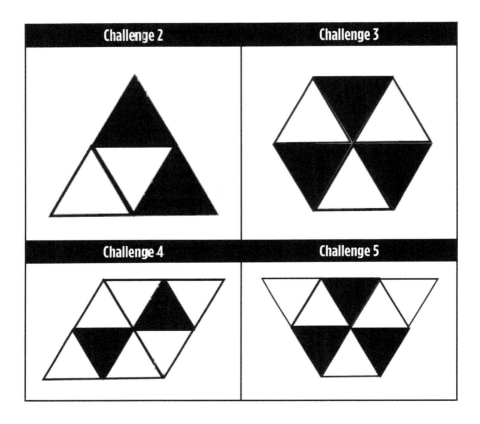

34—More Fractions

Say—I am going to show you some shapes. Be attentive and memorize them.

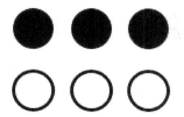

Ask the following questions.

Recall

How many circles in total? 6 circles

How many are black? 3 circles

How many are white? 3 circles

Manipulation

What is the fraction of the black circles? One-half

What is the fraction of the white circles? One-half

More examples

35-Find the Missing Number

Say–I am going to show you an equation. Be attentive and memorize it.

Challenge 1

$$3 + \text{\_\_\_} = 10$$

Ask the following questions.

Recall

Say the equation – 3 plus blank equals 10

Manipulation

What is the missing number? The missing number is 7

More examples

Challenge 2	Challenge 3
$5 + \rule{2em}{0.4pt} = 14$	$\rule{2em}{0.4pt} + 8 = 15$
Challenge 4	**Challenge 5**
$\rule{2em}{0.4pt} + 7 = 13$	$6 + \rule{2em}{0.4pt} = 16$

Note: You can do this activity with multiplication.

$$3 \times \rule{2em}{0.4pt} = 12$$
$$6 \times \rule{2em}{0.4pt} = 18$$
$$\rule{2em}{0.4pt} \times 4 = 24$$
$$\rule{2em}{0.4pt} \times 7 = 28$$

36–Area and Perimeter

Say–I am going to show you a shape. Be attentive and memorize it.

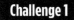

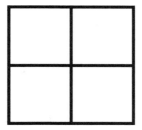

Ask the following questions.

Recall

How many squares? 4 squares

Manipulation

If each side of the little squares is one inch long, what is the perimeter? 8 inches

What is the area? 4 square inches

More examples

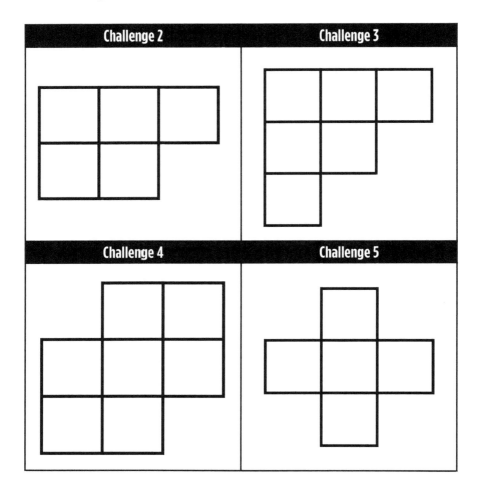

37-Nouns and Verbs

Say–I am going to read a sentence to you. Be attentive and memorize it.

Challenge 1

The boy ran with the dog.

Ask the following questions.

Recall
Repeat the sentence – The boy ran with the dog.

Manipulation
What is the verb? The verb is *ran*

What is the subject? The subject is *boy*

What was the last word in the sentence? The last word in the sentence is *dog*.

Note: You can read a sentence of any text and ask questions. Make a wise selection of which sentence to use.

More examples

Challenge 2

The girl jumped the rope.

Challenge 3

The cat scratched the sofa.

Challenge 4

The dog ate the bone inside the house.

Challenge 5

The squirrel hid the nut in the ground.

38-Rhyming Words

Say–I am going to read a sentence to you. Be attentive and memorize it.

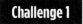

The duck is driving a truck

Ask the following questions.

Recall

Repeat the sentence – The duck is driving a truck.

Manipulation

What are the rhyming words? The rhyming words are *duck* and *truck*.

More examples

Challenge 2
Is that bug in my mug?

Challenge 3
A mouse is in my house.

Challenge 4
The lime cost a dime.

Challenge 5
She smells the rose with her nose

39–Letter Patterns

Say—I am going to show you some letters. Be attentive and memorize them.

Challenge 1

BABAB

Ask the following questions.

Recall

Say the pattern - BABAB

Manipulation

Mention the following three letters in the pattern - ABA

More examples

Challenge 2	Challenge 3
BBAAB	EGEGE

Challenge 4	Challenge 5
QQKKQ	XYYXY

40-Elapsed Time

Place students with a partner. One partner is A and the other is B.

Ask students to memorize what is under their letter.

Say–I am going to show you some times. Be attentive and memorize them.

Challenge 1

A	B
2:30 a.m.	**5:30 p.m.**

Ask the following questions

Recall
Repeat your time – 2:30 a.m. and 5:30 p.m.

Manipulation
How much time elapsed from one to the other? The elapsed time is 15 hours.

More examples

Challenge 2	
A	B
11:45 A.M.	9:45 P.M.
Challenge 3	
A	B
2:15 A.M.	8:15 P.M.
Challenge 4	
A	B
6:22 A.M.	1:22 P.M.
Challenge 5	
A	B
8:14 A.M.	6:14 P.M.

41-Money with Partners

Place students with a partner. One partner is 1 and the other is 2.

Ask students to memorize what is on their number.

Say–I am going to show you some money. Be attentive and memorize the coins.

Challenge 1

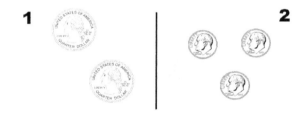

Ask the following questions.

Recall
Say your money – 2 quarters and 3 dimes

Manipulation
Add the coins together – 80 cents

Double the amount – $1.60

More examples

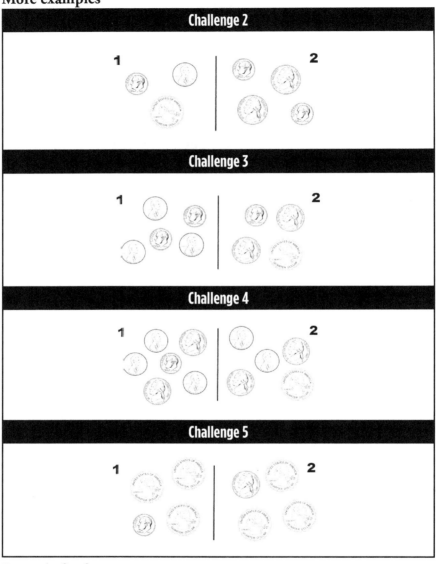

Example for four participants.

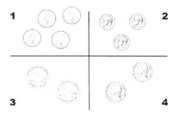

42-Letter Rotation

Say–I am going to show you some letters. Be attentive and memorize them.

Challenge 1

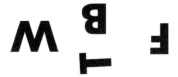

Take away the letters and then show the next ones.

Ask the following questions.

Recall

While showing the second set of letters, ask: What letters have stayed from the previous set? F and W

Manipulation

Which letters were added? T and B

How did the letters change in position? F and W rotated two times

Note: in this activity, students need to find out which letters were presented before. In addition, they have to inhibit distracting information as the new letters included.

More examples

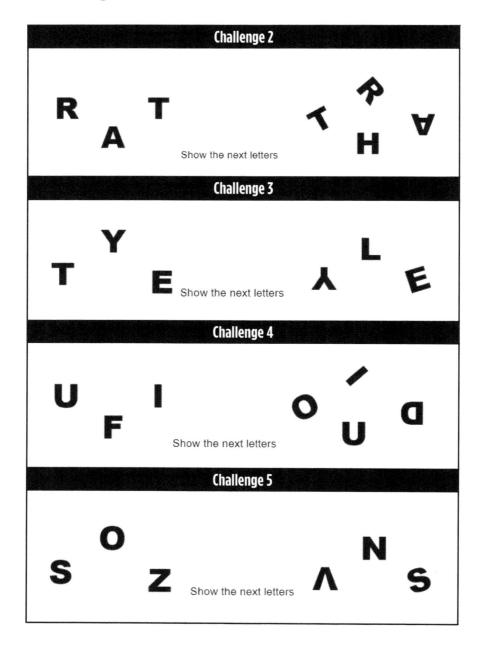

43–Shape Rotation

Say–I am going to show you some shapes. Be attentive and memorize them.

Challenge 1

Take away the shapes and then show the next ones.

 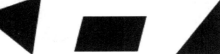

Ask the following questions.

Recall
While showing the second shapes, ask: What shapes stayed from the previous group? The two triangles

Manipulation
Which shape was added? The parallelogram was added.

How did the shapes change in position? The triangles rotated.

More examples

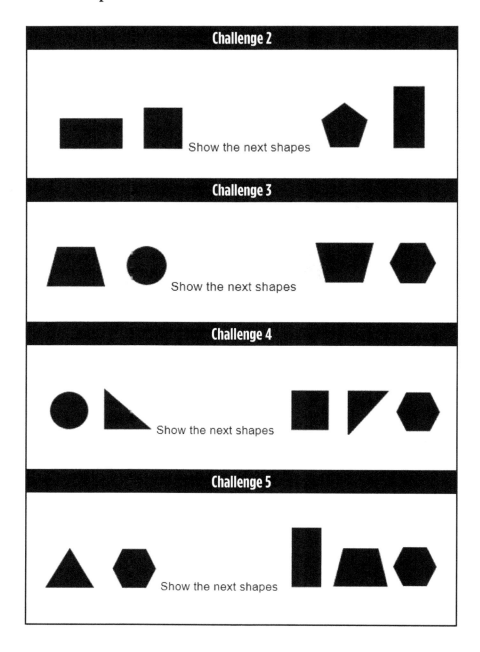

Challenge 2

Show the next shapes

Challenge 3

Show the next shapes

Challenge 4

Show the next shapes

Challenge 5

Show the next shapes

44-Prime and Composite Numbers

Say—I am going to show you a number. Be attentive and memorize it.

Challenge 1

245

Ask the following questions.

Recall

Say the number - 245

Manipulation

If you separate each number by itself:

What are the prime numbers? 2 and 5 are prime numbers.

What are the composite numbers? 4 is a composite number.

More examples

Challenge 2	Challenge 3
324	586

Challenge 4	Challenge 5
728	437

45–Forward and Backward with Numbers

Say–I am going to show you a number. Be attentive and memorize it.

Challenge 1

246

Ask the following questions.

Recall

Say the numbers - 246

Manipulation

Say the numbers backward – 6, 4, and 2

Say the second number – the second number is 4

More examples

Challenge 2	Challenge 3
369	468

Challenge 4	Challenge 5
975	753

46–Shape Patterns

Say–I am going to show you some shapes. Be attentive and memorize them.

Ask the following questions.

Recall

Say the pattern – circle, square, circle, square, and circle

Manipulation

Say the next shape in the pattern – square

More examples

47-Number Patterns

Say—I am going to show you some numbers in a pattern. Be attentive and memorize them.

3, 6, 9

Ask the following questions.

Recall

Say the numbers – 3, 6, and 9

Manipulation

Say the next two numbers in the pattern - 12, 15

More examples

Challenge 2	Challenge 3
18, 21, 24	24, 26, 28

Challenge 4	Challenge 5
12, 18, 24	15, 20, 25

48–Double the Black Number and Add the Other

Say–I am going to show you two numbers. Be attentive and memorize them.

$$10 \qquad 4$$

Ask the following questions.

Recall
Say the numbers: 10 and 4

Manipulation
Say the color of the numbers: 10 is gray, 4 is black

Double the black number: 4 x 2 = 8

Then, add the doubled number and the other number. 8 + 10 = 18

More examples

Challenge 2	Challenge 3
8 6	12 8

Challenge 4	Challenge 5
15 6	8 15

49-Odd and Even Numbers

Say–I am going to show you a number. Be attentive and memorize it.

Challenge 1

679

Ask the following questions.

Recall

Say the numbers - 679

Manipulation

Mention the odd numbers – 7 and 9

Mention the even numbers - 6

More examples

Challenge 2	Challenge 3
258	864

Challenge 4	Challenge 5
273	812

50-Moving Numbers with Two Digits

Say—I am going to show you some numbers. Be attentive and memorize them.

Challenge 1

54

Ask the following questions.

Recall

Say the number - 54

Manipulation

Move the first digit to the end. What number do you have now? I have the number 45.

More examples

Challenge 2	Challenge 3
72	48
Challenge 4	**Challenge 5**
98	57

51–Moving Numbers with Three Digits

Say–I am going to show you some numbers. Be attentive and memorize them.

Challenge 1

472

Ask the following questions.

Recall
Say the numbers - 472

Manipulation
Move the first digit to the end. What number do you have now? I have the number 724.

After you moved the number, move the first number again. What number do you have now? I have the number 247.

More examples

Challenge 2	Challenge 3
742	483

Challenge 4	Challenge 5
948	379

52–Alphabetical Order with Three-Letter Words

Say–I am going to show you a word. Be attentive and memorize it.

Challenge 1

PLY

Ask the following questions.

Recall

Say the letters - P, L, Y.

Manipulation

Order the letters in alphabetical order - L, P, Y.

More examples

Challenge 2	Challenge 3
TIE	TOE

Challenge 4	Challenge 5
VAN	WAR

53-Alphabetical Order with Four Letter Words

Say–I am going to show you a word. Be attentive and memorize it.

CAKE

Ask the following questions.

Recall
Say the letters: C, A, K, E.

Manipulation
Order the letters in alphabetical order - A, C, E, K.

More examples

Challenge 2	Challenge 3
HEAT	IDEA
Challenge 4	Challenge 5
KING	PAGE

WORKING MEMORY LESSON PLAN TEMPLATE

Skill/Say:_____

Challenge 1

Recall

Manipulation Questions

Increase difficulty in challenges

Challenge 2	Challenge 3
Challenge 4	Challenge 5

100 Numbers to Recall Chart

Use a number or more every day to challenge recall. When finished, create your own.

1. Show the number
2. Cover the number
3. Ask students to recall
4. Repeat the process with another number

1-12	21-667	41-4560	61-5500789	81-345006700
2-34	22-889	42-5670	62-6600899	82-456007800
3-56	23-231	43-6780	63-00112234	83-567008900
4-67	24-342	44-7890	64-11223345	84-001230045
5-89	25-453	45-11234	65-22334456	85-002340056
6-13	26-564	46-22345	66-33445567	86-004560078
7-45	27-675	47-33456	67-44556678	87-005670089
8-86	28-786	48-44567	68-55667789	88-010203040
9-78	29-897	49-55678	69-66778890	89-020304050
10-43	30-908	50-66789	70-12300456	90-030405060
11-123	31-1123	51-77890	71-23400567	91-040506070
12-234	32-2234	52-123450	72-34500678	92-050607080
13-456	33-3345	53-234560	73-45600789	93-060708090
14-567	34-4456	54-345670	74-112233456	94-0010020034
15-678	35-5567	55-456780	75-223344567	95-0020030045
16-789	36-6678	56-567890	76-334455678	96-0030040056
17-119	37-7789	57-1100123	77-445566789	97-0040050067
18-223	38-8890	58-2200234	78-556677890	98-0050060078
19-445	39-2340	59-3300456	79-123004500	99-0060070089
20-556	40-3450	60-4400678	80-234005600	100-1002003004

Bibliography

Ackerman, P. L., Beier, M. E., & Boyle, M. O. (2005). Working memory and intelligence: The same or different constructs? Psychological Bulletin, 131, 30-60.

Ackerman, P. L., Beier, M. E., & Boyle, M. O., (2005). Working memory and intelligence: The same or different constructs? Psychological Bulletin, Vol. 131. 30-60.

Adams, J. W., & Hitch, G. J. (1997). Working memory and children's mental addition. Journal of Experimental Child Psychology, 67, 21-38. Article No. CH972397.

Alloway, T. P. (2006). How does working memory work in the class-room? Educational Research and Review, Vol. 1 (4), pp. 134-139.

Alloway, T. P., & Alloway, R. G. (2010). Investigating the predictive roles of working memory and IQ in academic attainment. Journal of Experimental Child Psychology, 106, 20-29.

Alloway, T. P., & Gathercole, S. E. (2006). How does working memory work in the classroom? Educational Research and Reviews, Vol. 1 (4), 134-139.

Alloway, T. P., Gathercole, S. E., & Elliot, J. (2009). The cognitive and behavioral characteristics of children with low working memory. Child Development, Vol. 80, No. 2, 606-621.

Alloway, T., & Alloway, R. (2013). The Working memory advantage; Train your brain to function stronger, smarter, faster. New York. Simon & Schuster.

Archer, A. L., & Hughes, C. A. (2011). Explicit instruction; Effective and efficient teaching. New York: Guilford Press.

Atkinson, R.C., & Shiffrin, R. M. (1968). Human memory: a proposed system and its control processes. The Psychology of Learning and Motivation: Advances in Research and Theory. Vol. 2, 89-195.

Atkinson, R.C., & Shiffrin, R. M. (1971). The control of short-term memory. Scientific American. 225, 82-90.

Baddeley et al. (1986). Dementia and working memory. Quarterly Journal of Experimental Psychology, 38A, 603-618.

Baddeley et al. (1988). When long-term leaning depends on short-term storage. Journal of Memory and Language, 27, 586-595.

Baddeley et al. (1998). The phonological loop as a language learning device. Psychological Review, Vol. 105, 158-173.

Baddeley, A. (1993). Your memory; A user's guide. London. Penguin Group.

Baddeley, A. D., & Logie, R. (1999) Working memory: The multiple component model. In: Models of working memory: Mechanisms of active maintenance and executive control, ed. A. Miyake & P. Shah. Cambridge University Press.

Baddeley, A. D., Hitch, G. J., & Allen, R. J. (1993). Working memory and binding in sentence recall. Journal of Memory and Language, 61, 438-456.

Baddeley, A., Vallar, G., & Wilson, B. (1987). Sentence comprehension and phonological memory: Some neuropsychological evidence. In M. Coltheart (Ed.), Attention and performance 12: The psychology of reading, p. 509–529.

Ball et al. (2002). Effects of cognitive training interventions with older adults: a randomized controlled trial. J Am Med Assoc, 288(18), 2271–81.

Ball et al. (2013). Speed of processing training in the ACTIVE study: how much is needed and who benefits? J Aging Health, 25, 65S–84S.

Bherer (2008). Transfer effects in task-set cost and dual-task cost after dual-task training in older and younger adults: Further evidence for cognitive plasticity in attentional control in late adulthood. Exp Aging Res. 34(3), 188-219.

Bjorklund, D.F., & Douglas, R.N. (1997). The development of memory strategies. In N. Cowan (ed.), The development of memory in childhood, 201–246. Hove : Psychology Press

Blom, E., Küntay, A. C., Messer, M., Verhagen, J., & Leseman, P. (2014). The benefits of being bilingual: Working memory in bilingual Turkish-Dutch children. Journal of Experimental child Psychology, 128, 105-119.

Brophy, J., & Good, T., (1986). Teacher-effects results. In M.C. Wittrock (Ed.), Handbook of research on teaching, 3rd Edition, 328–375. New York: Macmillan.

Bui et al. (2013). The roles of working memory and intervening task difficulty in determining the benefits of repetition. Psychon Bull Rev, 20, 341-347.

Bull, R., & Scerif, G. (2001). Executive functioning as a predictor of children's mathematics ability: Inhibition, switching, and working memory. Developmental Neuropsychology, 19(3), 273-293.

Buonomano, D. (2011). Brain bugs; How the brain's flaws shape our lives. New York. W. W. Norton & Company, Inc.

Cain et at. (2004) Children's reading comprehension ability: Concurrent prediction by working memory, verbal ability, and component skills. Journal of Educational Psychology, Vol. 96, 31-42.

Cattell, R. B. (1963). Theory of fluid and crystallized intelligence: A critical experiment. Journal of Educational Psychology, 54(1), 1–22.

Chein, J. M., & Morrison, A. B. (2010). Expanding the mind's workspace: Training and transfer effects with a complex working memory span task. Psychonomic Bulletin & Review, 17(2), 193-199.

Chevalier et al. (2012). Underpinnings of the cost of flexibility in preschool children: The roles of inhibition and working memory. Dev Neuropsychol, 37(2), 99-118.

Cowan et al. (1992). The role of verbal output time in the effects of word length on immediate memory. Journal of Memory and Language, 31, 1-17.

Cowan N, Saults J. S., Elliott, E. M., & Moreno, M. (2002). Deconfounding serial recall. Journal of Memory and Language, 46(1), 153–177.

Cowan, N., (2014). Working memory underpins cognitive development, learning, and education. Educ Psychol Rev, 2(2), 197-223.

De Jong, P. F. (1998). Working memory deficits of reading disabled children. Journal of Experimental Child Psychology, 70, 75–96.

De Jong, T., & Van Joolingen, W. R. (1998). Scientific discovery learning with computer simulations of conceptual domains. Review of Educational Research, 68, 179–201.

Dempster, F. N. & Corkill, A. J. (1999). Interference and inhibition in cognition and behavior: Unifying themes for educational psychology. Educational Psychology Review, 11, 1-88.

DeStefano, D., & LeFevre, J. A. (2004). The role of working memory in mental arithmetic. European Journal of Cognitive Psychology, 16, 353-386.

Doidge, N. (2007). The brain that changes itself: Stories of personal triumph from the frontiers of brain science. New York. Penguin Books.

Dosher, B. A., & Ma, J.-J. (1998). Output loss or rehearsal loop? Output-time versus pronunciation-time limits in immediate recall for forgetting-matched materials. Journal of Experimental Psychology: Learning, Memory, and Cognition, 24(2), 316–335.

Dumontheil. I., Klingberg, T. (2012). Brain activity during a visuo-spatial working memory task predicts arithmetical performance 2 years later. Cereb Cortex, 22(5), 1078–1085.

Duncan, J., Mortiz, S., Thompson, R., & Dumontheil, I. (2012). Task rules, working memory, and fluid intelligence. Psychon Bull Rev, 19, 864-870.

Duncan, J., Schramm, M., Thompson, R., & Dumontheil, I. (2012). Task rules, working memory, and fluid intelligence. Psychon Bull Rev, 19, 864-870.

Eagleman, D. (2011). Incognito; The secret lives of the brain. New York. Vintage Books.

Ebbinghaus, H. (1964). Memory; A contribution to experimental psychology. New York. Dover Publications.

Engel de Abreu, P. M. J., Gathercole, S. E., & Martin, R. (2011). Disentangling the relationship between working memory and language: The roles of short-term storage and cognitive control. Learning and Individual Differences, 21, 569–574

Ericsson, A. (1991). The study of violinists at the music academy of West Berlin is published in one of the most seminal papers in the study of expertise: K. Anders Ericsson, Ralf Th. Krampe, and Clemens Tesch-Romer (1993). "The role of deliberate practice in the acquisition of expert performance. Psychological Review, no. 3, 363-406.

Furst, F. J., & Hitch, G. J. (2000). Separate roles for executive and phonological components of working memory in mental arithmetic. Memory and Cognition, 28 (5), 774-782.

Gardiner, J. M., Gawlik, B., & Richardson-Klavehn, A. (1994). Maintenance rehearsal affects knowing, not remembering: elaborative rehearsal affects remembering, not knowing. Psychonomic Bulletin & Review. 1(1), 107-110.

Gathercole, S. E., & Adams, A.-M. (1993). Phonological working memory in very young children. Developmental Psychology, 29(4), 770–773.

Gathercole, S. E., & Alloway, T. P. (2008). Working memory and learning: A practical guide for teachers. Sage Publication, 50.

Gathercole, S. E., & Hitch, G. J. (1993). Developmental changes in short-term memory: A revised working memory perspective. In A. Collins, S. E. Gathercole, M. A. Conway, & P. E. Morris (Eds.), Theories of memory (pp. 189-210). Hillsdale, NJ: Erlbaum.

Gathercole, S. E., Adams, A.-M., & Hitch, G., (1994). Do young children rehearse? An individual-differences analysis. Memory & Cognition, 22(2), 201-207.

Gathercole, S. E., Alloway, T. P., Kirkwood, H. J., Elliott, J. G., Holmes, J., & Hilton, K. (2008). Attentional and executive function behaviors in children with poor working memory. Learning and Individual Differences, 18, 214-223.

Gathercole, S. E., Elliott, J. & Alloway, T. P. (2008). Identifying and supporting children with poor working memory. Dyslexia Review, 19, 4-8.

Gathercole, S. E., Hitch, G. J., Service, E., & Martin, A. J. (1997). Phonological short-term memory and new word learning in children. Developmental Psychology, 33(6), 966-979

Gathercole, S. E., Lamont, E., & Alloway, T. P. (2006). Working memory in the classroom. In S. Pickering (Ed.), Working memory and education, 219–240.

Gathercole, S. E., Pickering, S. J., Ambridge, B., & Wearing, H. (2004). The structure of working memory from 4 to 5 year of age. Developmental Psychology, Vol. 40. No 2, 177-190.

Gathercole, S. E., Willis, C. S., Baddeley, A. (2004). The structure of working memory from 4 to 5 year of age. Developmental Psychology, Vol. 40. No 2, 177-190.

Gathercole, S.E, & Alloway, T. P. (2004). Working memory and classroom learning. Dyslexia Review, 15, 4 – 9.

Gathercole, S.E, & Alloway, T. P. (2006). Working memory deficits in neurodevelopmental disorders. Journal of Child Psychology and Psychiatry, 47, 4 – 15

Gathercole, S.E, & Alloway, T.P. (2008). Working memory and learning: A practical guide. London: Sage Publications.

Geary, D. C. (1990). A componential analysis of an early learning deficit in mathematics. Journal of Experimental Child Psychology, 49, 363–383.

Gernsbacher, M. A., (1993). Less skilled readers have less efficient suppression mechanisms. Psychol Sci, 4(5), 294-298.

Gersten, R., Schiller, E. P., & Vaughn, S. (2000). Contemporary special education research. Mahwah, NJ: Erlbaum.

Goldstein, J. M., Jerram, M., Poldrack, R., Anagnoson, R., Breiter, H. C., Makris, N., Goodman, J. M., Tsuang, M. T., & Seidman, L. J. (2005). Sex differences in prefrontal cortical brain activity during fMRI of auditory verbal working memory. Neuropsychology, 19, 509–519.

Green, C. S., & Bavelier, D. (2003). Action video game modifies visual selective attention. Nature, 423, 534-537.

Guthrie, J. T. (2004). Teaching for literacy engagement. Journal of Literacy Research, 36, 1-28.

Hasselmo, M. E., & Stern, C. E. (2006). Mechanisms underlying working memory for novel information. Trends Cogn Sci, 10(11). 483-493.

Hill et al. (2014). Gender differences in working memory networks: A brainmap meta-analysis. Biol Psychol., 18-29.

Hitch, G. J., & Schaafstal, A. M. (1988). Visual working memory in young children. Memory and Cognition, 28 (5), 774-782.

Holmes, J., Gathercole, S. E., & Dunning, D. (2009). Adaptive training leads to sustained enhancement of poor working memory in children. Dev. Sci, 12, F9–15.

Holmes, J., Gathercole, S. E., & Dunning, D. L. (2009). Adaptive training leads to sustained enhancement of poor working memory in children. The Authors Journal Compilation, Blackwell Publishing Ltd.

Holmes, J., Gathercole, S. E., & Dunning, D. L. (2010). Poor working memory: Impact and interventions. Advances in Child Development and Behavior, 39, 1-43.

Hughes, C. (1998). Finding your marbles: Does preschoolers' strategic behavior predict later understanding of mind? Developmental Psychology, 34(6), 1326–1339.

Jaeggi et al. (2008). Improving fluid intelligence with traning on working memory. Proceedings of the National Academy of Sciences of the United States of America, 105(19), 6829-6833.

Jensen, E. (1998). Teaching with the brain in mind. Alexandria, VA. Association for Supervision and Curriculum Development.

Jones, G. (2012). Why chunking should be considered as an explanation for developmental change before short-term memory capacity and processing speed. Frontiers in Psychology, Vol 3. 1-8

Kane et al. (2007). For whom the mind wanders, and when: An experience-sampling study of working memory and executive control in daily life. Psychological Science, Vol. 18, 614-621.

Kane, M. J., & Engle, R. W. (2002). The role of prefrontal cortex in working-memory capacity, executive attention, and general fluid intelligence: An individual-differences perspective. Psychonomic Bulletin & Review, 9, 637-671.

Kane, M. J., & Engle, R. W. (2002). The role of prefrontal cortex in working-memory capacity, exectutive attention, and general fluid intelligence: An individual-differences prespective. Psychonomic Bulletin & Review, 9(4), 637-671.

Kaufman, S. B. (2007). Sex differences in mental rotation and spatial visualization ability: Can they be accounted for by differences in working memory capacity? Intelligence, 35, 211–223.

Klingberg et al. (2002). Training of Working Memory in Children with ADHD. Journal of Clinical and Experimental Neuropsychology, Vol. 24. 781-791.

Klingberg, T. (2002). Training of working memory in children with ADHD. Journal of Clinical and Experimental Neuropsychology, Vol. 24, 781-791

Klingberg, T. (2009). The overflowing brain; Information overload and the limits of working memory. New York. Oxford University Press.

Klingberg, T. (2010). Training and plasticity of working memory. Trends Cogn. Sci, 14, 317–24.

Klingberg, T., Fernell, E., Olesen, P., Johnson, M., & Gustafsson, P. (2005). Computerized training of working memory in children with ADHD—a randomized, controlled trial. J. Am. Acad. Child Adolesc. Psychiatry, 44, 177–86.

Kyllonen, P. C., & Christal, R. E. (1990). Reasoning ability is (little more than) working-memory capacity? Intelligence, 14, 389-433.

Kyllonen, P. C., & Christal, R. E. (1990). Reasoning ability is (little more than) working-memory capacity. Intelligence, 14, 389-433.

Lejbak, L., Crossley, M., & Vrbancic, M. A. (2011). Male advantage for spatial and object but not verbal working memory using the n-back task. Brain and Cognition, 76, 191–196.

Lewin et al. (2001). Sex differences favoring women in verbal but not in visouspatial episodic memory. Neuropsychology, Vol. 15, 165-173.

Lynn, R., & Irwing, P. (2008). Sex differences in mental arithmetic, digit span, and g defined as working memory capacity. Intelligence, 36, 226–235

Maraver et al. (2016). Training on working memory and inhibitory control in young adults. Frontiers in Human Neuroscience, Vol 10. 1-18.

Marchand-Martella, N., Blakely M. & Schaefer, E. (2004). Aspects of schoolwice implementations. In N. Marchand-Martella, Slocum,

T., & Martella, R. (Eds.), Introduction to direct instruction, 304-331. Boston: Pearson.

Masters, M. S., & Sanders, B. (1993). Is the gender difference in mental rotation disappearing? Behavior Genetics, 23, 337-341.

McLean, J. F., & Hitch, G. J., (1999). Working Memory Impairments in Children with Specific Arithmetic Learning Difficulties. Journal of Experimental Child Psychology, 74, 240-260.

McLeod, P., & Posner. M. I. (1984). Privileged loops from percept to act. In H.Bouma & D.G.Bouwhuis (Eds.), Attention and performance X: Control of language processes. Hove. UK: Lawrence Erlbaum Associates Ltd.

Miller, G. A. (1956). The magical number seven, plus or minus two: Some limits on our capacity for processing information. Psychological Review, 63, 81–97.

Moher, M., Tuerk, A, S., & Feigenson, L. (2012). Seven-month-old infants items in memory. J Exp Child Psychol, 112(4), 361-377.

Morales, J., Calvo, A., & Bialystok, E. (2012). Working memory development in monolingual and bilingual children. J Exp Child Psychol, 114 (2), 187-202.

Nation, K., Adams, J. W., Bowyer-Crane, C. A., & Snowling, M. J. (1999). Working memory deficits in poor comprehenders reflect underlying language impairments. Journal of Experimental Child Psychology, 73, 139–158.

Nordvik, H., & Amponsah, B. (1998). Gender differences in spatial abilities and spatial activity among university students in an egalitarian educational system. Sex Roles, 38, 1009–1023

Oei et al. (2006). Psychosocial stress impairs working memory at high loads: An association with cortisol levels and memory memory retrieval. Stress, 9(3), 133-141.

Ottem et al. (2007). Reasons for the growth of traditional memory span across age. European Journal of Cognitive Psychology, 19, 233-270.

Passolunghl et al. (2013). Mathematics anxiety, working memory, and mathematics performance in secondary-school children. Frontiers in Psychology, Vol 7. 1-8.

Pavlov, I. (1849-1936), Classical Conditioning. Retrieve from: https://www.learning-theories.com/classical-conditioning-pavlov.html

Pearson et al. (2014). Working memory retrieval as a decision process. Journal of Vision, 14(2):2, 1-15.

Pennington, B.F, and Oxonoff, S. (1996). Executive functions and developmental psychopathology. Journal of Child Psychology and Psychiatry, 37, 51-87.

Pianta et al. (2007). Opportunities to learn in america's elementary classrooms. Science, 315(5820). 1795-1796.

Postle, B., R. (2012). Activation and information in working memory research. The Wiley-Blackwell Handbook on the Cogn. Neuroscience of memory.

Quartz, S., R. and Sejnowski, T., J. (2002). Liars, lovers, and heroes; What the new brain science reveals about how we become who we are. New York. HarperCollins Publishers, Inc.

Repovs, G., & Baddeley, A. D. (2006). The multi-component model of working memory: explorations in experimental cognitive psychology. Neuroscience, 139, 5-21.

Restak, R. M. (1979). The brain; The last frontier. Garden City, NY. Boubleday & Company.

Restak, R. M. (1991). The brain has a mind of its own; Insights from a practicing neurologist. New York. Harmony Books.

Restak, R. M. (1995). Brainscapes; An introduction to what neuroscience has learned about the structure, function, and abilities of the brain. New York. Hyperion.

Restak, R. M. (2001). Mozart's brain and the fighter pilot; Unleashing your brain's potential. New York. Harmony Books.

Restak, R. M. (2001). The secret life of the brain. New York. The Dana Press and the Joseph Henry Press.

Restak, R. M. (2003). The new brain; How the modern age is rewiring your mind. Rodale. www.rodalestore.com.

Restak, R. M. (2009). Think smart; A neuroscientist's prescription for improving your brain's performance. New York. Riverhead Books.

Restak, R. M. (2010). The playful brain; The surprising science of how puzzles improve your mind.

Reynolds, G. D., & Romano, A. C. (2016). The development of attention systems and working memory in infancy. Frontiers in Systems Neurosicence, 1-12.

Riley, M. R., & Constantinidis, C. (2016). Role of prefrontal persistent activity in working memory. Frontiers in Systems Neuroscience, Vol. 9, 1-14.

Ripley, A. (2013). The smartest kids in the world. New York: Simon & Schuster.

Rodriguez et al. (2000). Engaging Texts: Effects of Concreteness on Comprehensibility, Interest, and Recall in Four Text Types. Journal of Educational Psychology, Vol. 92, 85-95.

Rosenshine, B. (1997) 'The Case for Explicit, Teacher-Led, Cognitive Strategy Instruction', paper presented at the annual meeting of the American Educational Research Association, Chicago, IL, March.

Rosenshine, B., & Stevens, R. (1986). Teaching functions. In M. C. Wittrock (Ed.), Handbook of research on teaching, 3rd Edition, 376-391. New York: Macmillan.

Rotzer, S., Loenneker, T., Kucian, K., Martin, E., Klaver, P., & Von Aster, M. (2009). Dysfunctional neural network of spatial working memory contributes to developmental dyscalculia. Neuropsychologia, 47, 2859-2865.

Salamé, P., & Baddeley, A. D. (1982). Disruption of short-term memory by unattended speech: Implications for the structure of working memory. Journal of Verbal Learning & Verbal Behavior, 21(2), 150–164.

Salthouse, T. A. (1994). The aging of working memory. The american psychological association.

Schmiedek et al. (2010). Adult age differences in covariation of motivation and working memory performance: Contrasting between-person and within-person findings. Research in Human Development, 7(1), 61-78.

Schneiders, et al. (2012). The impact of auditory working memory training on the fronto-parietal working memory network. Frontiers in Human Neuroscience, Vol 6. 1-14.

Schoofs, D., Wolf, O. T., & Smeets, T., (2009). Cold pressor stress impairs performance on working memory tasks requiring executive functions in healthy young men. Behavioral Neuroscience, Vol 123. 1066-1075.

Service, E. & Craik, F. I. M.(1993). Differences between Young and Older Adults in Learning a Foreign Vocabulary. Journal of Memory and Language, 32, 608-623.

Service, E. & Kohonen, V. (1995). Is the relation between phonological memory and foreign language learning accounted for vocabulary acquisition? Applied Psycholinguistics, 16, 155-172.

Shields et al. (2016). The effects of acute stress on core executive functions: A meta-analysis and comparison with cortisol. Neurosci Biobehav Rev, 68. 651-668.

Shields, G. S., Bonner, J. C., & Moons, W. G. (2015). Does cortisol influence core executive functions? A meta-analysis of acute cortisol administration effects on working memory, inhibition, and set-shifting. Psychoneuroendocrinology, 58, 91–103.

Shields, G. S., Sazma, M. A., & Yonelinas, A. P. (2016). The effects of acute stress on core executive functions: A meta-analysis and comparison with cortisol. Neuroscience and Biobehavioral reviews, 68, 651–668. http://doi.org/10.1016/j.neubiorev.2016.06.038

Shields, G. S., Sazma, M. A., & Yonelinas, A. P., (2016). The effects of aucte stess on core executive functions: A meta-analysis and comparison with cortisol. Neurosci Biobehav Rev, 68, 651-668.

Siegel, L. S., & Ryan, E. B., (1989). The Development of Working Memory in Normally Achieving and Subtypes of Learning Disabled Children. Child Development, 60, 973-980.

Simmering, V. R., & Perone, S. (2013). Working memory capacity as a dynamic process. Frontiers in Psychology, 1-26.

Simmons, D. C., Fuchs, L. S., Fuchs, D., Mathes, P., & Hodge, J. P. (1995). Effects of explicit teaching and peer tutoring on the reading achievement of learning disabled and low-performing students in the classroom. The Elementary School Journal, 95, 387–408.

Smeekens, B. A., & Kane, M. J. (2016). Working memory capacity, mind wandering, and creative cognition: An individual-differences investigation into the benefits of controlled versus spontaneous thought. Psychol Aesthet Creat Arts, 10(4). 389-415.

Smith, S., & Pichora-Fuller, M. K. (2015). Associations between speech understanding and auditory and visual test of verbal working memory: Effects of linguistic complexity, task, age, and hearing loss. Frontiers in Psychology, Vol 6. 1-15.

Smolen, T., & Chuderskl, A. (2015). The quadratic relationship between difficulty of intelligence test items and their correlations with working memory. Frontiers in Psychology, Vol 6. 1-13.

St Clair-Thompson, H., & Holmes, J. (2008). Improving short-term and working memory: Methods of memory training. Nova Science Publishers, Inc.

Stanley et al. (2014). Changes in global and regional modularity associated with increasing working memory load. Frontiers in Human Neuroscience, Vol 8. 1-14.

Stroop, J. R., (1935). Studies of Interference in serial verbal reactions. Journal of Experimental Psychology, Vol. 18, No. 6.

Stuss, D. T., & Alexander, M. P. (2000). Executive functions and the frontal lobes: a conceptual view. Pyschological Research. 63, 289-298.

Stuss, D.T., & Alexander, M. P. (2000). Executive functions and the frontal lobes: A conceptual view. Psychological Research, 63, 289-298.

Swanson, H. L. (1999). What develops in working memory? A life span perspective. Developmental Psychology, 35(4), 986–1000.

Swanson, H. L. (2015). Cognitive strategy interventions improve word problem solving and working memory in children with math disabilities. Frontiers in Psychology, Vol 6. 1-13.

Swanson, H. L., & Berninger, V. (1995). The role of working memory in skilled and less skilled readers' comprehension. Intelligence, 21, 83– 108

Swanson, H. L., & Sachse-Lee, C. (2001). Mathematical problem solving and working memory in children with learning disabilities: Both executive and phonological processes are important. Journal of Experimental Child Psychology, 79, 294–321.

Swanson, L., & Kim, K. (2007). Working memory, short-term memory, and naming speed as predictors of children's mathematical performance. Intelligence, 35, 151–168.

Thorell, et al. (2008). Training and transfer effects of executive functions in preschool children. Developmental Science, 11(6), 969-976.

Towse, J. N., Hitch, G. J., & Hutton, U. (1998). A reevaluation of working memory capacity in children. Journal of Memory and Language, 39, 195-217.

Tulving E., & Patkau, J. E. (1962). Concurrent effects of contextual constraint and word frequency on immediate recall and learning of verbal material. Canadian Journal of Psychology, 16(2), 83–95.

Tulving et al. (2005), The oxford handbook of memory. Oxford & New York: Oxford University Press.

Tulving, E. (1983). Elements of Episodic Memory. Oxford: Clarendon Press.

Tulving, E. (2001). 'Episodic memory and common sense: how far apart?' Phil. Trans. R. Soc. Lond. B., 356, 1505-1515.

Tulving, E. (2002). 'Episodic memory: From mind to brain'. Annual Review of Psychology, 53, 1-25.

Tulving, E., & Schacter, D. (1990). Priming and human memory systems. Science, Vol. 247, 301–306.

Tulving, E., (1972). Episodic and semantic memory. In Organization of memory of memory (ed. E. Tulving and Donaldson). 381-403.

Tulving, G. E., & Pearlstone, Z. (1966). 'Availability versus accessibility of information in memory for words'. Journal of Verbal Learning and Verbal Behavior, 5, 4, 381-391.

Unsworth et al. (2015). Working memory and fluid intelligence: Capacity, attention control, and secondary memory retrieval. Cogn Psychol, 71, 1-26.

Valenzuela et al. (2003). Memory training alters hippocampal neurochemistry in healthy elderly. Neuropsychiatric Institute, Vol 14, No 10.

Van Dyke et al. (2014). Low working memory capacity is only spuriously related to poor reading comprehension. Cognition, 131(3), 373-403.

Westerberg, H., & Klingberg, T. (2007). Changes in cortical activity after training of working memory – a sigle-subject analysis. Physiology & Behavior. Karolinska Institutet, Department of Neuropediatircs. Stockhom, Sweden.

Wilhelm, O., Hildebrandt, A., & Oberauer, K. (2013). What is working memory capacity, and how can we measure it? Frontiers in Psychology, Vol 4. 1-22.

Wilson, K. M., & Swanson, H. Lee. (2001). Are mathematics disabilities due to a domain-general or a domain-specific working memory deficit? Journal of Leaning Disabilities, Vol. 34, No. 3.

Wimmer et al. (2000). The double-deficit hypothesis and difficulties in learning to read a regular orthogrphy. Journal of Educational Psychology. Vol. 92, 668-680.

Wykes, T., Brammer, M., Mellers, J., Bray, P., Reeder, C., Williams, C., & Corner, J. (2003). Effects on the brain of a psychological treatment—cognitive remediation therapy: functional magnetic resonance imaging in schizophrenia. Br J Psychiatry, 181, 144-152.

CPSIA information can be obtained
at www.ICGtesting.com
Printed in the USA
LVHW021329160423
744469LV00031B/574